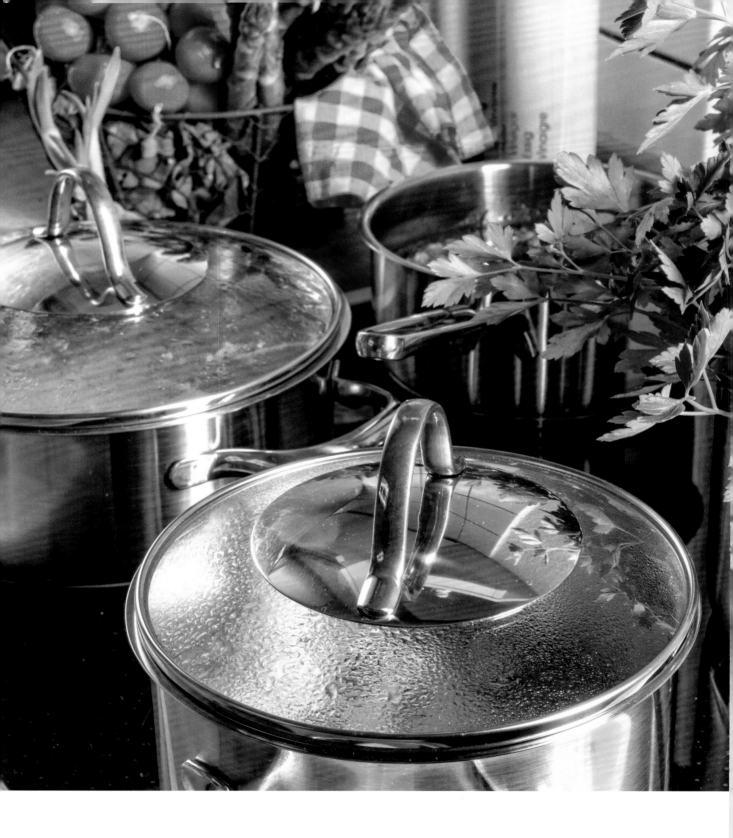

INTRODUCTION

I have always had a "love-hate" relationship with food. Having first been diagnosed with disordered eating at the age of 19, I became well familiar with in-patient treatment, psychologists and psychiatrists, and licensed social workers. Yet nothing really helped for the long haul until I became enamored with the art of cooking. Where behavioral modifications, antidepressants, and group therapy failed, learning how to cohesively *craft* a meal—along with how food can strengthen (or erode) our mental and physical health—proved to be the path of healing I'd been seeking for more than two decades.

Exploring the creative process of eating was a complete game changer for me in regards to my health, plus my career. The origin and quality of the ingredients, complementary beverage pairings, and food styling techniques all impact our overall dining experience—whether at home or in a five-star establishment. I've been able to merge the practical knowledge I've soaked up as a culinary writer over the last ten years with all the expertise I gained in the fitness industry as an instructor and mindfulness practitioner. Thus, the next natural step for me was becoming a Certified Holistic Nutritionist. Food can *(and should be)* a source of beauty, wellness, and delight in our lives. And I am thrilled you've decided to join me on this journey to de-stress eating...the *macro* way.

Maybe you've heard all the buzz about #IIFYM (If It Fits Your Macros). And maybe you're skeptical, which is reasonable. Having the flexibility to eat foods you enjoy more often than on an occasional "cheat day" sounds too good to be true. But that is exactly why macro-based nutrition *does* work. Satiety doesn't get left by the wayside—nor does your sanity. Freedom from obsessing over every bite comes from leaning into what nosh builds you up versus what leaves you tapped out...or in a persistent state of hunger. *Figuring out the right balance of carbs, protein, and fat for your body is going to release you from dieting.*

So what does that freedom look like, and how do you achieve it? I'll show you in the pages that follow. First, I'll explain what macros are and what makes a macro-eating plan so optimal for the human body. Then, I'll show you how to figure out the right ratio of these nutrients that is best suited to your individual health goals. I'll also give you plenty of tips and advice for easing into the macro-based lifestyle. Finally, you and I are going to manifest well-being via the joy-*fullness* that can be a part of every meal. I'll share with you some of my favorite recipes that will help kickstart your macros journey.

So come join me in the kitchen. We've got plenty of cooking—and tasting—to do!

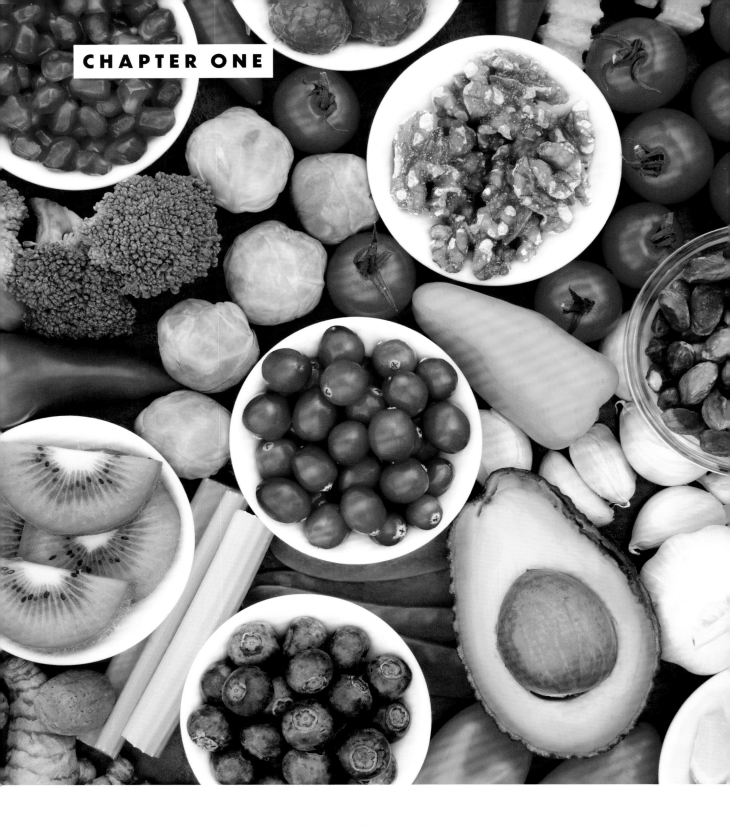

CHAPTER ONE

WHY MACRO?

Nourishment: a buzz word that rolls easily off the tongue but a concept that can be much more difficult to attain in our daily lives. Finding the right foods to support your physical—and mental—health is an evolving process, a reality most fad diets fail to acknowledge. What is adequate nutrition today could be deficient in terms of sufficiently fueling your body, and mind, even a few months from now.

I personally struggled with this reality for nearly twenty years. My relationship with food felt like a dysfunctional domestic partnership: constantly shifting dynamics that always led back to square one—being out of balance in terms of time spent and tangible positive outcomes. My nutritional preferences over the years have ranged from being *vegan* to *pescatarian*, in addition to a few clinically unhealthy eating patterns. I always seemed to be consuming too much or too little. The concept of moderation did not seem achievable until I started learning how to approach wellness from a more holistic perspective.

While working in the fitness industry as a trainer, instructor, and model for almost ten years, I would come to discover that my story is not an unusual one. Even when you're committed to making intentional choices to improve—as well as maintain—your health, figuring out the right combination of *functional foods* to stay on track can feel like a jigsaw puzzle you were never meant to solve. Especially since overly processed grub tends to be the cheapest available.

This fact, along with our perpetual lack of time to prepare "from scratch" home-cooked meals, enables the diet industry to generate over $255 billion in profits annually worldwide. So if eating "right" is a perpetual moving target, does any reliable information exist to properly assess our dietary intake? Luckily, the core of our cellular makeup provides an ideal blueprint through its reliance upon *macronutrients*.

Pescatarian: A dietary plan that is heavily plant-based plus integrates fish and seafood.

Vegan: A dietary lifestyle that eliminates animal by-products in all forms. This includes meat, poultry, seafood, eggs, all dairy products, and for some, honey as well.

Vegetarian: Also sometimes called *lacto-ovo vegetarian*, a nutritional preference based on abstaining from eating meat, yet still incorporates eggs or dairy products into meals.

Flexitarian: A dietary plan that is plant-based most of the time, but may occasionally include meat or fish.

Functional foods: Foods that may have a positive effect on health beyond basic nutrition by supporting optimal body conditioning and helping to lower the risk of disease (when consumed on a regular basis and at certain levels).

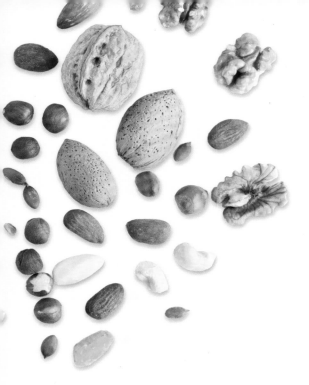

HIDDEN DANGERS
OF A POOR DIET

Inadequate nutrition can have dire health consequences long term—regardless of gender, race, ethnicity, socioeconomic status, or country of residence. A poor diet either lacks healthy foods or contains too many unhealthy foods; either way, poor diet can increase the risk of dying prematurely. Research conducted by the Global Burden of Disease Study on how diet affects lifespan additionally found that worldwide, we are eating:

- 12% of the recommended amount of nuts and seeds
- 16% of the recommended amount of milk
- 23% of the recommended amount of whole grains
- 90% more processed meat than is recommended
- 86% more sodium than is recommended
- 18% more red meat than is recommended

THE SCIENCE BEHIND MACRONUTRIENTS

Macronutrients are the three basic components of food: carbohydrates, protein, and fat. According to Julie Andrews, R.D., a nutritionist and creator of The Healthy Epicurean, macros are the primary nutrients that give us energy because, combined, they represent the number of calories we consume daily. "The amount a person needs of each macronutrient and total calories differs depending on their age, gender, height, weight, activity level, etc.," she says. "But all three macros perform different and important functions in the body related to metabolism, hormones, and more."

Andrews emphasizes the importance of understanding that most foods contain more than one macro, and it's essential to balance all three. "If a recipe happens to be a low source of one of the macros, I'll suggest a pairing to go with the recipe to complete the meal," she says. For example, you could add grilled salmon to a vegetable and bean salad to be sure you're getting adequate protein, making this meal "macro complete." Andrews also aims to include "high-quality sources of macronutrients," which means the food provides other essential nutrients such as fiber, vitamins, and minerals.

"If a recipe includes a source of fat (like olive oil and salmon), as well as a source of carbohydrates (like beans, vegetables, and nuts or seeds) in addition to a source of protein (thanks to the beans and salmon), it's providing a host of benefits," Andrews says. "Think omega-3s from the salmon; fiber from the beans and vegetables; vitamin E from the olive oil; a host of other vitamins and minerals from the vegetables...the list goes on."

Although obtaining this macronutrient trio that Andrews notes can be done easily enough, the specific amounts of each one you consume should directly align with your individual health goals—shifting when needed as different priorities emerge or the next phase of life begins. So, what exactly does each macronutrient do?

MACROS 101

The human body needs specific nutrients to function properly. Our cells can't sufficiently produce energy, minimize inflammation, maintain gut health, facilitate metabolism, and stabilize blood sugar if a state of inadequate nutrition is the norm. Understanding how food has the capacity to catalyze, as well as sustain, wellbeing begins with understanding the basics behind all our nutritional needs—the macros.

Carbohydrates

Carbs are the primary energy source for our bodies since they all, with the exception of fiber, are converted into sugar (also known as glucose). Recent diet trends have made this vital source of human fuel out to be the villain. In reality, carb intake, when properly portioned, can be a potent energy source rather than a detriment in terms of helping to stave off cravings and fatigue.

"Carbohydrates are important for fueling the brain, central nervous system, and red blood cells," says Andrews. And if the carbohydrate source is high quality—that is, it contains fiber—it can "aid digestion and help you feel fuller, longer."

Vary the type of carbs you eat as much as time and budget will allow. Rice and potatoes might be two of the cheapest staples to craft meals around. However, the more you mix it up, the more versatile your micronutrient intake will be. Try to also hone in on any physical and/or mental sensations that arise in the first three to four hours after eating—any brain fog, lethargy, discomfort, etc. For example, although I don't have celiac disease, I eat pasta only about twice a month because consuming more than a few servings of gluten-containing foods within a week triggers a noticeable amount of bloating for me.

Another reason carbs get a bad rap is the energy spike and crash that things such as sweets and refined products like white bread can cause. High-quality carbs, on the other hand, are "more slowly digested, keeping you fuller," notes Andrews. "They do not cause as much of a spike

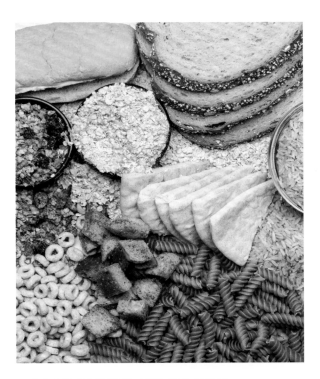

CARBOHYDRATE FOODS

- Grains
- Whole grains*
- Fruits*
- Vegetables*
- Beans*
- Legumes*
- Milk (lactose)
- (*contains fiber)

and drop of your blood sugar, which can make you irritable and hungry, and cause cravings." Every gram of carbohydrate is 4 calories.

Protein

Constant cravings may be a sign your current protein intake is too low. Our bodies use more calories to metabolize protein than other types of food because it accounts for 20 percent of the average person's body weight. Water is the only substance that accounts for a higher proportion of the human body's physical composition than protein.

"Proteins consist of amino acids that build and repair tissues and muscles in the body; provide structure to cells, organs, hair, skin, and nails;

PROTEIN FOODS

- Meat
- Poultry
- Smoked turkey breast*
- Roast skinless chicken breast*
- Egg whites*
- Seafood
- Cod fillets*
- Prawns*
- Canned light tuna*
- Salmon*
- Nuts and seeds
- Beans*
- Legumes*
- Lentils*
- Dairy products
- Greek yogurt*
- Soy products
- Tofu*
- Tempeh*
- Seitan

(*Lean protein)

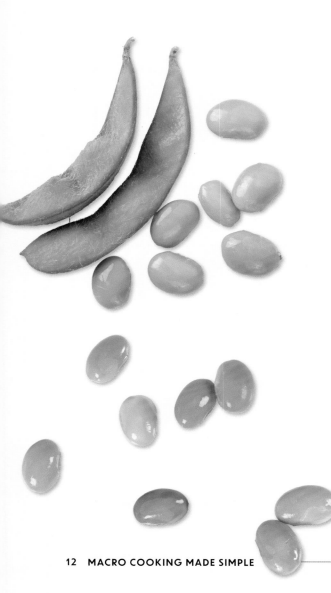

maintain the body's pH level; and create enzymes and hormones necessary for bodily functions," explains Andrews.

The average recommended daily protein intake for adults is 1 gram of protein per kilogram of body weight. This amount may slightly increase during times of illness, surgery recovery, or advanced age. Although this dietary requirement can be met by eating many plant- or animal-derived foods, in order to avoid unnecessarily increasing the risk of developing heart disease or certain types of cancer, try to meet your target level for this macro with *lean protein* sources such as smoked turkey breast, canned light tuna, lentils, and Greek yogurt. While you don't need to eliminate non-lean protein options altogether, lean protein is your healthier bet. Every gram of protein is 4 calories.

Raw nuts are one of my primary snack foods specifically because they're a quick source of protein that's easy to carry, plus they have a decent shelf life when stored properly. I'll munch on a handful periodically throughout the day or add a few tablespoons to meals whenever and however I can. I also really appreciate how many different kinds there are. Tired of eating almonds? Switch to cashews, walnuts, or pecans for a bit. A close friend once told me I eat like a "healthy squirrel." I continue to take that as a compliment.

As for protein powders and bars: If you are eating an adequate amount of each macro, these items are better used as supplemental nutrition to help you stay on track during long work shifts, road trips, international travel, or backpacking excursions.

> **Lean protein:** The US Department of Agriculture (USDA) defines lean protein as less than 10 g fat, 4.5 g or less saturated fat, and less than 95 mg cholesterol per 3.5 ounces (100 g).

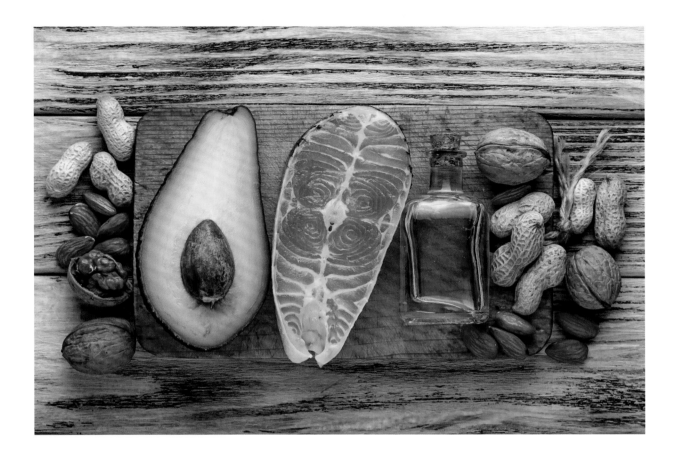

Fat

Food myths abound regarding fat. What amount is *too much* or *too little* seems to be constantly debatable. However, one proven fact is fat (just like carbs and protein) is necessary to help cells fully utilize the foods we eat.

"Fats help your body absorb fat-soluble vitamins (A, D, E and K), are responsible for storing energy, and help the body insulate organs," says Andrews. "We need a variety of fat-containing foods to keep us healthy."

Although the different types of fat are not interchangeable, having too much of one and not enough of another can negatively affect your health. So knowing the difference between *trans fat*, *saturated fat*, *unsaturated fat*, and *fatty acids* is key. Every gram of fat, regardless of type, is 9 calories.

Trans fat: The two types of trans fats associated with food are *naturally occurring* and *artificial*. Naturally occurring trans fats are produced in the gut of some animals, and the foods made from these animals (like beef, buttermilk, and lamb) might have small amounts. In contrast, artificial trans fats are the partially hydrogenated oils found in many processed foods because it is cheap to produce and significantly reduces food spoilage. Some restaurants and fast-food chains also use trans fats to deep-fry foods because oils containing it can be reused in commercial fryers.

The problem with trans fats is that too much can increase "the bad" (LDL) cholesterol levels and lower "the good" (HDL) cholesterol levels. If you're looking to lower your risk of developing type 2 diabetes or cardiovascular issues, start phasing out mass-produced, pre-packaged pizzas, cookies, cakes, pies, microwave popcorn, and margarine. Look for words like "hydrogenated" and "partially hydrogenated oil" on food labels as a clue.

Saturated fat: These fat molecules are solid at room temperature, like butter or the fat on a well-marbled steak. Most saturated fats are consumed as meat and other animal products, like eggs and whole-fat dairy, plus some tropical plant sources such as coconut, palm oil, and palm kernels. A diet too high in saturated fat can also elevate LDL and total cholesterol levels, two factors known to contribute to heart disease.

Unsaturated fat: Unsaturated fat exists in two forms: *monounsaturated*, which has only one double bond between carbon molecules, and *polyunsaturated*, which has two or more double bonds. Usually liquid at room temperature, both increase HDL cholesterol levels in the blood, which can positively impact heart health. Common sources of unsaturated fats include avocados, olives, salmon, almonds, pistachios, pecans, pine nuts, and walnuts, in addition to some oils like safflower, sunflower, and olive.

***Essential* fatty acids:** There are two types of polyunsaturated fatty acids (omega-6 and omega-3), which are considered to be "essential" because they can't be made by the human body to sustain itself. This means our only way of ensuring we get the amount needed for the vital functions they support is through adequate nutrition. Foods that contain omega-6 include seeds and seed oils like sunflower, hemp, and sesame, in addition to nuts and nut oils like walnuts; corn, wheat germ, soybeans, poultry, and some dairy products also contain omega-6s. Omega-3s are most readily accessible through fish, eggs, and seaweed. Other potential sources are dark-green vegetables such as broccoli and spinach, flax and chai seeds, canola oil, walnuts, and butternuts.

UNCOUPLING FAT AND SODIUM

A lot of high-fat foods come with high sodium levels as well. But they need not go hand-in-hand. If a low-sodium lifestyle is a priority for you, these swaps are a cinch to execute in the kitchen:

- Use low-sodium chicken or veggie broth as a partial (or full) replacement for oil in most entrée recipes. Bonus: this trick decreases the total fat amount too.
- To make a dish more savory while keeping sodium levels at bay, try using light miso paste, kelp, low-sodium tamari, or celery salt.
- Don't underestimate the flavor punch of acids, such as lemon juice and vinegar, or herbs such as dill or basil.

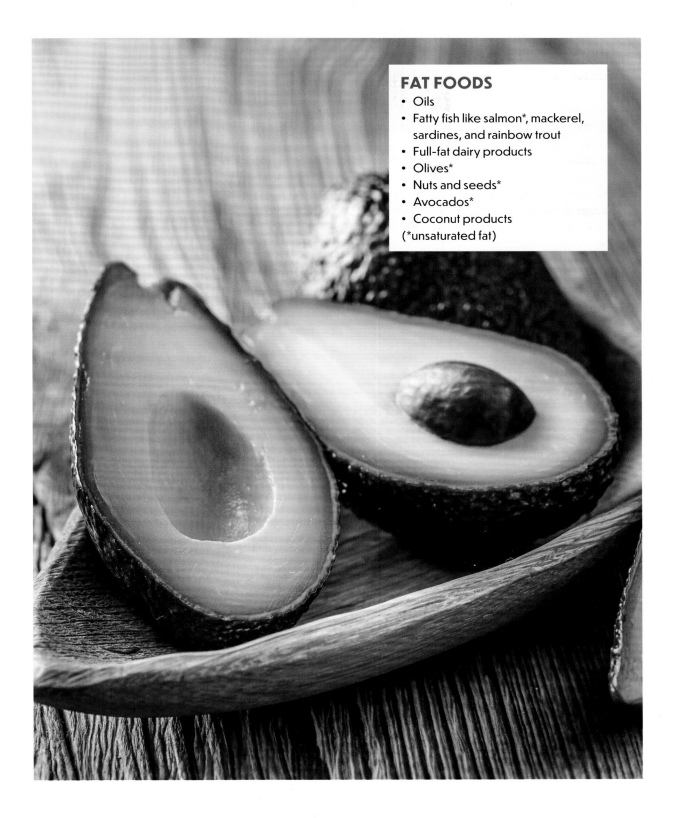

FAT FOODS

- Oils
- Fatty fish like salmon*, mackerel, sardines, and rainbow trout
- Full-fat dairy products
- Olives*
- Nuts and seeds*
- Avocados*
- Coconut products

(*unsaturated fat)

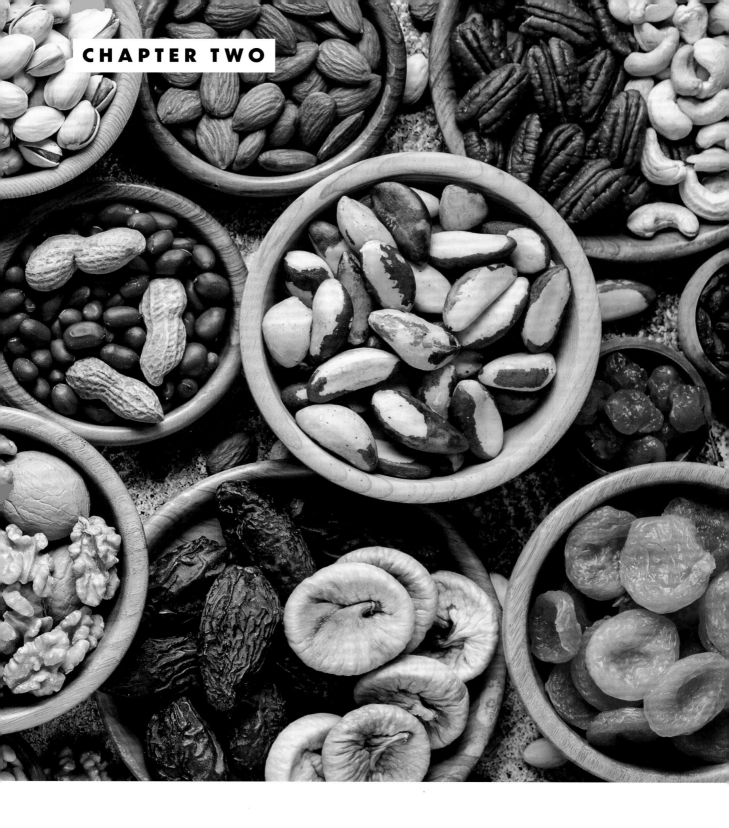

CHAPTER TWO

LIVING THE MACRO LIFE

Now that you have the nitty-gritty about what the macros are, I hope you can see that one of the *best* parts about a macro-centered approach to eating is the *flexibility*. Plant-based, keto, paleo, gluten-sensitive, low sodium...all dietary preferences are welcome here! As long as carb, protein, and fat portions are calculated correctly, being an omnivore or herbivore, or having food allergies, doesn't put you at a significant disadvantage.

WHAT'S IN & WHAT'S OUT?

Every photo in this book is meant to spark a feeling of inspiration, rather than restriction. Being healthy and enjoying food and beverages were never meant to be mutually exclusive! But you might have other questions about what's "allowed" on a macro-centric eating plan, and I have some answers.

Can I still have my coffee, or do I have to start drinking less?
That depends on how much coffee you drink daily, on average. And *why*. Having an espresso or latte is truly a fave moment for me on any given day, so I would be the first person to tell you to tap the caffeine freely if it was in your best interest. But in reality, the chronic fatigue you may often battle might be attributable to nutrient imbalance. If having two or more caffeinated beverages in a 24-hour period is the norm, test out scaling back; see if you can use a midday stroll, or an earlier bedtime, to ward off afternoon slumps.

Are snacks allowed?
Absolutely! Eating is meant to be a pleasurable experience, not puritanical. If you do not genuinely enjoy many of the foods you normally eat, the time has come to discover ones you do, because a nutritious nosh shouldn't feel punitive or insufficient. So if—based on your fitness routine, academic schedule, career demands, or family obligations—snacks ensure you're energized to tackle the day's "to do" list, don't cut them out. Simply assess whether there are healthful alternatives, like Pumpkin Oat Bars (page 131) or Matcha Gems (page 123), that increase endurance thanks to key ingredients the body can run off for a longer period of time—as opposed to the big sugar spike, then rapid crash, many processed foods induce.

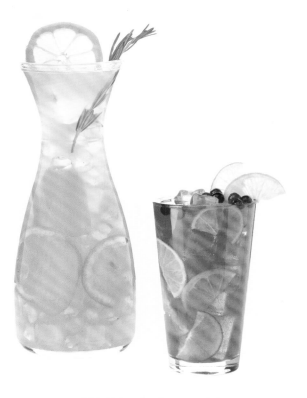

MORE "DRY LIFE" ADVICE, COURTESY OF DR. LIIA RAMACHANDRA

- Alcohol dehydrates you. When your body is dehydrated, it can lead to very dry and irritated skin and faster aging. That puffiness and redness in your face is due to dehydration.
- Alcohol is also known to disrupt your sleep. The skin and body regenerate the most during the night; therefore, if sleep is disrupted, the regeneration and restoration either slows or does not happen.
- Drink lots and lots of water before, during, and after drinking alcohol. Natural juices such as tomato and celery are great as well because they contain vitamins that encourage liver detoxification.
- Improve circulation and detoxification in your body through exercises such as yoga and walking.

Can I drink alcohol?

The short answer is yes, but a good course of action is to reduce consumption if you habitually have more than five to seven drinks a week. Also, spend some time reflecting on whether your patterns of imbibing are bringing you closer to, or pushing you farther away from, the healthy lifestyle you seek.

For example, I've drastically cut back on when (and how) much I drink, and I'm actively working toward eliminating booze altogether. I needed to get honest about the complete lack of health benefits alcohol has for me. As an avid runner, I would like to continue competing in races for as long as possible. I'm also a certified yoga instructor, so sweating out the adult beverages I had the night before really doesn't aid me in showing up on my mat fully present.

One of the repeated comments I hear from friends when opting to abstain at social functions is how they can appreciate my motivation but would never personally do it because they just want to "enjoy their lives." Except, in many ways, I am relishing my life now more than ever before. I can't say I miss the hangovers, spotty memory, and sluggish workouts that inevitably tagged along each morning after. My guess is you probably wouldn't either...so why not give it a try during the next Dry January or Sober October? Consider journaling along the way to track any notable struggles and successes. Mix up my Low-Cal Lassi recipe (page 149) to get started on a tasty note. Added bonus is it looks just as chic on camera—or social media—as any frozen boozy cocktail.

Do I need to cut out sugar?

This is where we pause to take a deeper dive into your personal pleasure philosophy. For so many of us, the concept of "treating ourselves" is associated with decadent dinners, gourmet chocolate, and/or drinkable sugar bombs (aka, fruity cocktails). But once "self-care" is detached from edible goods, how much sugar you are "allowed" becomes less about *quantity* and more about *intent*.

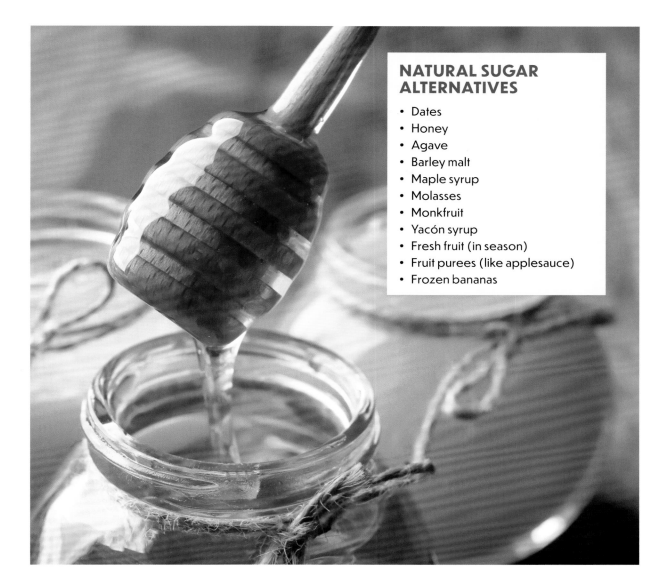

NATURAL SUGAR ALTERNATIVES

- Dates
- Honey
- Agave
- Barley malt
- Maple syrup
- Molasses
- Monkfruit
- Yacón syrup
- Fresh fruit (in season)
- Fruit purees (like applesauce)
- Frozen bananas

For example, having dessert multiple nights a week might be low-key comforting. However, cuddle time with a partner/child/pet, a massage twice a month, or taking an extended weekend once a quarter to hike, travel, or merely sleep in will soothe your whole being. When the next urge for sweet treats emerges, before reconfiguring your macro count, think about whether there is anything else you could add to this month's *pleasure program* that would uplift you even more.

Do I have to cut out all processed foods?
No. Nor is processed food the villain you need to be constantly vigilant of when trying to adhere to a macro-nutritional plan. Case in point: I eat primarily plant-based, so a fair amount of the proteins I consume are meat substitutes. Same goes for the dairy-free cheeses and yogurts stocked in my fridge. You can't "milk" a cashew, thus there's no denying that these items are processed. However, adding protein-dense, faux "chick'n" strips to stir-fry a couple times a week

is vastly different than habitually snacking on potato chips. If your choices consistently reflect quality over quantity, rest assured, you're likely being judicious about when and how to integrate processed foods into meals.

What, if any, supplements should I be taking to support my macro intake?

Even though many of us may have noticed the benefits of taking multivitamins, fish oil, or probiotics, it's wise to tread lightly with any supplement, herbal remedy, or micronutrient product. If you are meeting your macro needs sufficiently, it's unlikely you'll need additional supplementation. Plus, taking excess amounts of certain vitamins and minerals can be just as harmful as having a deficiency. Start by touching base with your primary health care provider or a complementary medicine specialist (such as a naturopathic doctor, registered dietitian, or a certified nutritionist) to review what prescriptions and over-the-counter meds you are already taking. It's extremely important to confirm none of the supplements you are wanting to add-in could decrease the effectiveness of a medication you are already on—or cause an adverse reaction—if taken too close together in the same day.

Do I have to eat more meat (or cut back on some of the meat)?

The ability to flex eating styles is one of the biggest adventures (and advantages) of macro cooking. If your nutrient ratio calls for a significant increase in protein, think of foods you have yet to try or would like an excuse to find fresh ways to prepare. Also don't feel pressured to do a complete overhaul of your recipe box overnight. If you're curious about cutting back on meat, it's perfectly reasonable to start by experimenting on Meatless

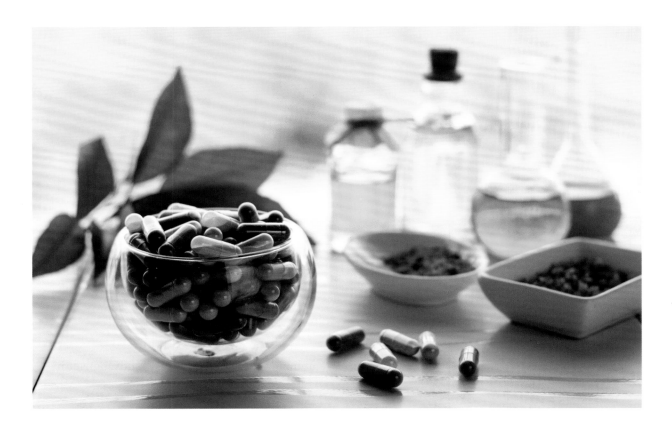

Mondays or participating in Veganuary come January. My Black Bean Tostadas on page 93, in particular, is a quick, flavorful entrée to whip up—and modify—regardless of whether you're feeling more like an herbivore or a carnivore these days.

MINDFUL EATING WITH MACROS

Hopefully, tweaking your cooking feels more exciting than overwhelming. Stress and eating are two words that don't really belong together. If you regularly feel anxious about your nutritional habits, either at home or on the go, let's explore how mindfulness may spark a fresh outlook on all the ways menu planning and food prep can be joy-*filled*.

When dining out, I know how to savor food, but being fully present when eating at home is a habit I've been striving to cultivate for years. Unfortunately, there is no shortcut. Learning how to eat more intuitively requires being tuned in to the physical and mental sensations you experience before, during, and after mealtimes. Which is why *cleansing*, *intermittent fasting*, and *intentional eating* aren't merely trends without substance. Each involves approaching your nutritional intake with an aim of detoxifying and regaining balance; they're effective approaches for reigniting a desire for wholesome sustenance after indulging one too many days on holidays, vacation, or business trips. (But don't worry—I'm not asking you to start fasting!)

You can train yourself to be more mindful while eating. It starts with becoming more aware of the ebb and flow of what you eat, how much, and when based on your activity level, hormonal shifts, and other physiological factors. What this looks like in practice involves conscious choices like:

- Eating sans watching TV, working, or scrolling through your phone.
- Noticing physical sensations of hunger as they arise.
- Expanding your awareness to the visual aesthetics of food. *(Is it photo-worthy?)*

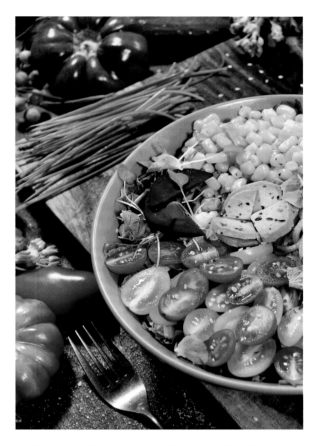

- Observing the aroma and colors of the food before digging in.
- Focusing on the texture, taste, and flavors you detect while chewing.
- Resting between bites, followed by taking a moment to notice any sensations or thoughts that come to mind. *(Do you have any discomfort? Tense facial expressions? Are you comfortable how and/or where you are seated?)*

Gradually, if we train ourselves to experience eating on a more holistic level, we'll improve our perception of fullness—thanks to employing each of the five senses at mealtimes. Train your mind to better perceive the sensuality of food and the act of eating. By approaching every table with an abundance mindset, it'll be a game changer in terms of staving off temptations that could derail your wellness journey.

Mindfulness: The practice of maintaining a nonjudgmental state of heightened or complete awareness of one's thoughts, emotions, or experiences in the present moment.

Food detox: Also known as *cleansing*, is a form of detoxification (that may involve fasting, teas, juices, or colonics) to trigger toxin release from the body. Detoxing can help boost metabolism, immunity, and overall health.

Intermittent fasting: Abstaining from eating (usually for a minimum of 12 hours, but no more than 40) multiple times a week or month. Water, black coffee or tea, and calorie-free drinks are usually permitted during the hours of fasting, but not any solid foods.

Intentional eating: A nutritional approach that brings together macro tracking and intuitive eating by fine-tuning one's awareness of the body's response as changes and fluctuations in food consumption occur. For example, if you are feeling hungrier after the first two meals of the day, intentional eating would mean adjusting your remaining macros to include more nutrient-dense items instead of ignoring body cues—or throwing off your tracking altogether by binging later in the evening.

FUELING YOUR BODY

Food choices should empower you, not leave you feeling less energetic—or guilt-ridden. And spending hours fretting over what you shouldn't be eating is far less important than allowing yourself to explore new patterns of nourishment. Yes, food is one pathway. But so is hydration. As is movement. Ideally, these lifestyle elements form a personalized health trifecta working together to nurture your body. But when one area is lacking, the whole system is thrown off balance. This negatively impacts the body's ability to fully process and absorb nutrients, in addition to sleep quality and mood stability. You feel drained because you are drained.

Is there one food that can fix all this? No. There also is not merely three or four. However, eating wholesome meals tailored to your ongoing needs is an accessible path to discovering an optimal state of wellbeing. One that *will* occasionally fluctuate. Yet, also one you will be much better equipped to navigate by having the knowledge to adjust macros accordingly during periods of illness, stress, or major life transitions.

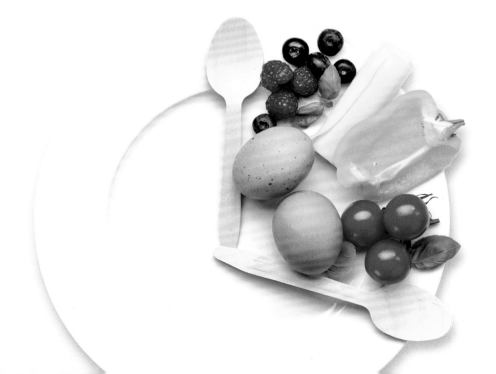

MACRO MINDSET MAP

I journal frequently to help center my mind as well as to gain clarity on which foods, people, and spaces aid or inhibit my ability to actualize my goals. Use your own notebook and the following prompts as a self-care guide reminding you to set aside time each week or month to reflect on the progress you're making.

What/who/where is helping to fuel you forward?

_____

_____

_____

What/who/where is a "mood bomb"? (e.g., negativity, anxiety, and/or stress trigger)

_____

_____

_____

This week, my "manifest" mantra is:

_____

_____

_____

One mindful moment I savored was:

_____

_____

_____

The next recipe I will make is:

_____

_____

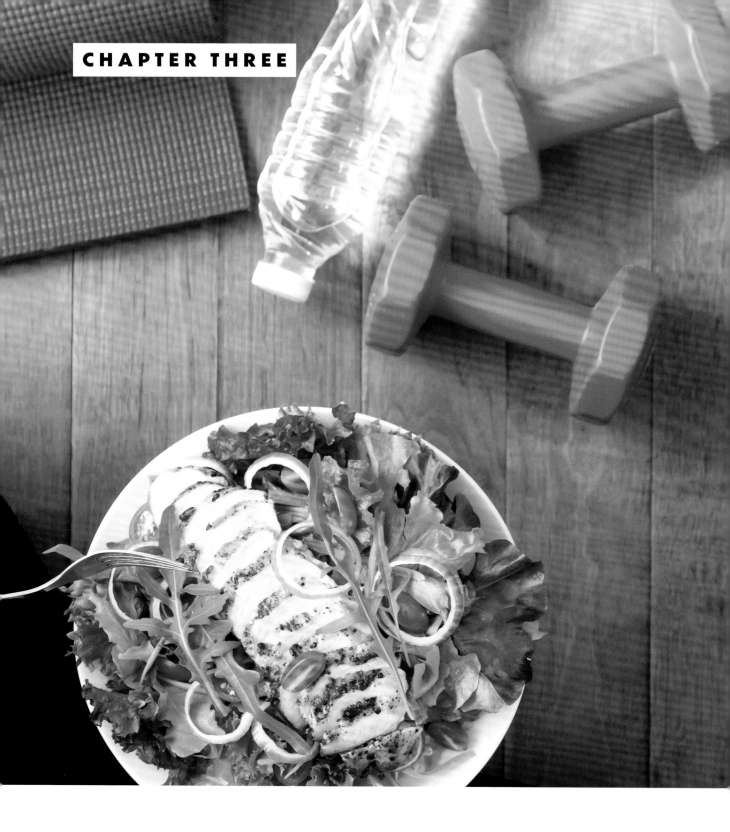

CHAPTER THREE

WORKING WITH YOUR MACROS

Now that you've had a crash course on the fundamentals of macro-based nutrition, this is the section where theory gets put to practical use. Before we get busy together in the kitchen, I'll break down the basics of determining macro ratios.

MACRO TRACKING VS. CALORIE COUNTING

Tracking macros and counting calories are often combined steps, but they are fundamentally different. When you solely focus on calorie amounts, it's usually because your desired outcome is weight loss. In theory, if you take in fewer calories than you burn, it should result in pounds dropped. The problem with this logic, however, is that a person can be skinny—and unhealthy. Body size is a faulty benchmark for assessing how well-nourished a person is.

This is why tracking macros can be enlightening in terms of how nutritious the meals you eat actually are. Three people of the same height and weight might all be eating the same number of calories in a day, but the macro breakdown of their individual diets would reveal more about who's actually more *fit*. Because it *does* matter where the calories come from in terms of nutritional breakdown, plus how the body puts that fuel to use.

Knowing the portions you consume (in grams or percentages) of proteins, carbs, or fats is the basis of macro-based nutritional plans. Many foods contain more than one macronutrient— yet another reason that increased awareness of your macro intake can be helpful if you have food allergies or sensitivities. Understanding food labels will become second nature thanks to paying closer attention to nutritional data and ingredients lists.

Of course, macro and calorie counting can both be problematic if it morphs into a person's only concern in terms of wellness. Regular exercise, as well as adequate sleep, also play a vital role in our health status. Avoid overly obsessing about what to—or not to—eat to the extent these other important factors get neglected.

Ultimately no matter the objectives you're working toward, monitoring macro ratios will allow you to adjust as needed, based on how hitting target levels is influencing your physical— and mental—health. Let's get started.

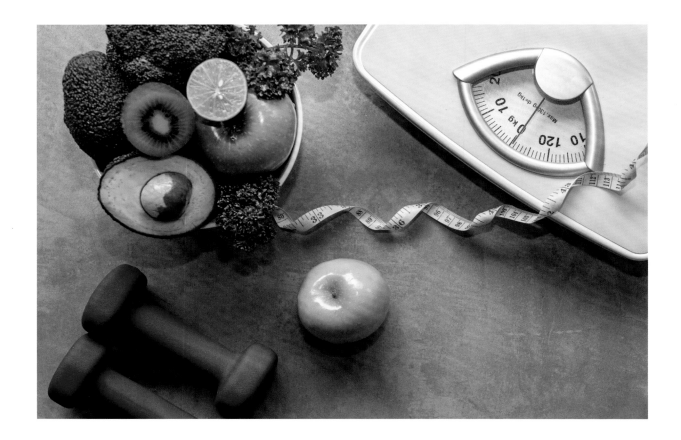

THE RATIO GUIDE: HOW TO VARY MACRO RATIOS FOR SPECIFIC HEALTH GOALS

This book is meant to be a nutritional compass to help identify the types of food—and their specific combinations—that will help you achieve, then maintain, the state of wellness you seek. If you're training for a marathon, your dietary intake needs will greatly differ than for someone who is recovering from surgery or who is still trying to regain their pre-quarantine level of fitness. Also keep in mind that what we eat does have the capacity to impact our moods as well. Modifying your choices of eats and drinks to better support mental health when dealing with chronic stress or depression is equally as important as keeping tabs on physical caloric needs.

You can craft a macro-focused nutrition plan to stimulate weight gain or fat loss. Or you can use it in weight maintenance or to acquire lean muscle mass. The National Academies of Science, Engineering, and Medicine recommends adults try to get 10 to 35 percent of their calories from protein, 45 to 65 percent from carbs, and 20 to 35 percent from fats. But as noted, individual macro ratios differ based on personal needs, so aside from working with a registered dietitian to guide you through the process, the easiest way to calculate a baseline macro range to get you going is with the Harris-Benedict equation. This is the macro amount you theoretically should already be consuming, calculated using your current weight and average level of physical activity:

Basal Metabolic Rate (BMR) x activity level = your Daily Amount of Calories (DAC)

---

1. DETERMINE BMR

Basal Metabolic Rate is the number of calories you burn each day with no physical activity. In other words, if you were on complete bed rest for 24 hours, this is how many calories your body would utilize.

To find your BMR, use this Mifflin–St. Jeor formula, which is an updated formula based on the original Harris-Benedict equation:

BMR for women

Metric:

BMR = (10 × weight in kg) + (6.25 × height in cm) − (5 × age in years) − 161

Imperial:

BMR = (4.536 × weight in pounds) + (15.88 × height in inches) − (5 × age) − 161

BMR for men

Metric:

BMR = (10 × weight in kg) + (6.25 × height in cm) − (5 × age in years) + 5

Imperial:

BMR = (4.536 × weight in pounds) + (15.88 × height in inches) − (5 × age) + 5

So, for example, a 43-year-old woman who weighs 158 pounds and is 5 feet 8 inches tall would have a baseline BMR of 1421, based on the following calculation:

(4.536 x 158) + (15.88 x 68) - (5 x 43) - 161 = 1421

And a 45-year-old man who weighs 180 pounds and is 6 feet tall would have a baseline BMR of:

(4.536 x 180) + (15.88 x 72) - (5 x 45) + 5 = 1739

Calculate your own BMR here:

_____

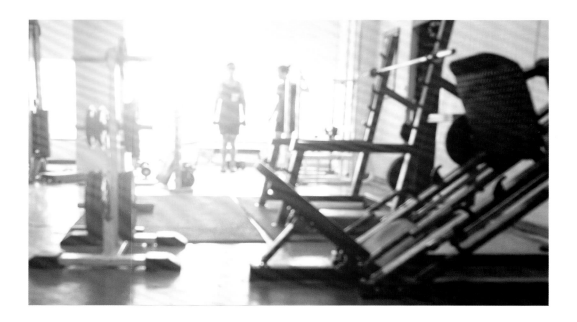

2. FACTOR IN CURRENT FITNESS REGIMEN

Exact macro ratios are set by multiplying BMR by how active you are on average, based on the following metrics:
- Little or no exercise: 1.2
- Light exercise a few times a week: 1.375
- Moderate exercise 3 to 5 times a week: 1.55
- Heavy exercise 6 to 7 times per week: 1.725
- Elite endurance training or strength conditioning: 1.9

Which means if the same woman from the previous example typically walks a few miles to work twice a week and attends three yoga classes, her moderate level of exercise results in an ideal DAC of 2202:

1421	x	1.55	=	2202
(BMR)		(activity level)		*(the number of calories she would aim to eat in a day for basic health maintenance)*

If the same man from the previous example typically runs five miles (8 km) three times a week, his moderate level of exercise results in an ideal DAC of 2695:

1739	x	1.55	=	2695
(BMR)		(activity level)		*(the number of calories he would aim to eat in a day for basic health maintenance)*

3. CHOOSE YOUR MACRO RATIO

Remember that every gram of protein and carbohydrate provides your body with 4 calories, while each gram of fat provides 9 calories. And calories are a measurement of supplied energy. The way you consume those calories—that energy—should reflect your health goals.

For example, to the right are the average macro ratios for some of popular dietary lifestyles. Based on your nutritional preferences, find your target ratios by multiplying the total baseline calories by the goal percentage of each food category. The protein and carbohydrate figures are then divided by 4 (*calories per gram*) and the fat figure by 9 (*calories per gram*).

Thus, if she was Paleo, the 2202-calorie baseline for our 43-year-old woman would break down in this macro ratio:

- Protein = 2202 (calories) x 0.45 (or, 45 percent) = 991/4 (calories per gram) = 248 g
- Carbohydrates = 2202 x 0.35 = 771/4 = 193 g
- Fat = 2202 x 0.2 = 440/9 = 49 g

OG Keto	
Protein	approx. 15%
Carbs	Less than 5% *(20 g or fewer, excluding fiber)*
Fat	approx. 80%

Low carb/high protein	
Protein	20% to 40%
Carbs	less than 5%
Fat	55% to 60%

Paleo	
Protein	45%
Carbs	35%
Fat	20%

Plant-based	
Protein	25% to 30%
Carbs	40% to 45%
Fat	30% to 35%

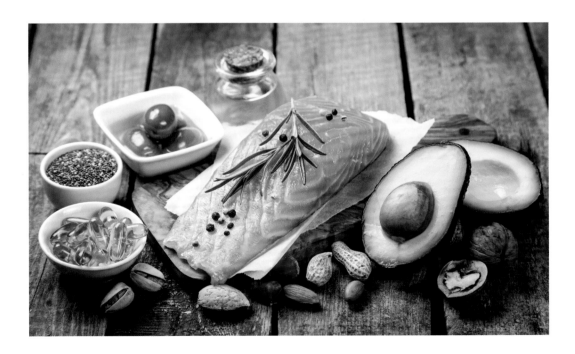

4. TWEAK TO SUIT YOUR WELLNESS GOALS

The beauty of following a macro-based eating plan is that you can also easily shift around your ratios to suit your shifting health goals and wellness needs. Because our lives aren't static, nor is what we eat, it's often more realistic to aim to land within a certain *range* for each macro, rather than feeling pressured to consistently hit one specific number. Here are some possible macro splits based on specific wellness objectives:

- For endurance training and/or competitive athletes, this ratio can enhance athletic performance: 40% to 45% carbs, 25% to 30% protein, and 30% fat.
- For weight loss, 40% to 50% protein, 20% to 30% carbs, and 20% to 30% fat is an appropriate starter range.
- For weight gain to improve health or for moderate to intense strength training 4 to 5 times a week: 40% to 60% carbs, 25% to 35% protein, and 15% to 25% fat.

It is also important to note the essential role protein plays in the formation and repair of muscle tissue. This is why most experts insist more protein is needed in order to gain muscle, as well as prevent loss. Thus, when in doubt, skewing your macro intake toward protein consumption (more than carbs and fat), combined with regular strength training, is most likely to spark muscle gain plus fat loss.

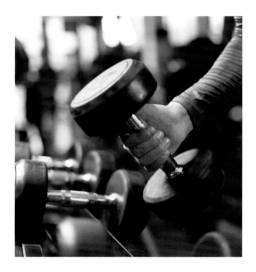

Yes, hitting the macro range you computed is a priority. It won't always be perfect, especially in the beginning—and that's okay. Give yourself time to experiment, while also modifying target ratios as you attain your goals. But here are some things you'll start to notice as you consistently follow your macro plan:

- Eating an adequate amount of protein should steadily start to manifest as increased muscle mass.
- Properly calculated carb intake should stabilize blood sugar enough so that you experience fewer random cravings throughout the day.
- Adding in healthy fats should progressively feel like second nature rather than a list of forbidden foods you're constantly trying to avoid.

5. HACK YOUR MACRO TRACKING

Don't stress out thinking you'll be forever crunching numbers. That's definitely not the end goal! You also shouldn't stress about trying to compute the macro ratio of individual meals or snacks. Aim to land within your target ranges cumulatively for the day. Meal prepping and menu planning is also another way to stick within the macro portions you've worked out—allowing you to pre-portion out your food for the week.

The reality is most of us have many demands on our time without the freedom to eat at home for every meal or take home-cooked meals with us wherever we go. I have a general idea of how my ratio is flowing as the day progresses. And I'll often flex my meals when it becomes apparent, say by midafternoon, that my intake is shaping up to leave me at a noticeable deficit in one area. Or I'll scale back if a restaurant meal ends up being more robust than I'd anticipated.

It's also not realistic to try to limit yourself to only foods that have nutrient info on a label. Fresh produce doesn't have those details mapped out; neither do meat cuts you order at the butcher or deli counter. Again, don't stress! Eventually, the IIFYM life will become second nature to you as well, so you'll gradually become less reliant on "doing the math."

For now, opt for digital assistance if frequently doing macro calculations is becoming too much of a time drain. One of the best components of several macro tracking apps is that they are useful in a wide variety of settings. Whether cooking at home, eating out with friends, or on vacation, you will have the info needed to *crunch numbers* easily accessible via your mobile device. Most apps request you input height, age, and activity level to calculate an ideal calorie range for the weight goals you specified. You can even preset macro percentages based on dietary preferences such as vegan, keto, paleo, etc. Go with your gut in terms of which app seems the most user friendly for you, plus one that is likely to fill a gap in terms of daily support for staying on track. For example, if you frequently travel for work or take clients to lunch, picking a tech tool that is loaded with dining-out data is a smart choice.

TRACKING APPS

Here are a few that have gotten great reviews, but there are many more out there.

- Carb Manager
- Cronometer
- LifeSum
- My FitnessPal
- My Macros+
- Macrostax
- Nutritionix Track

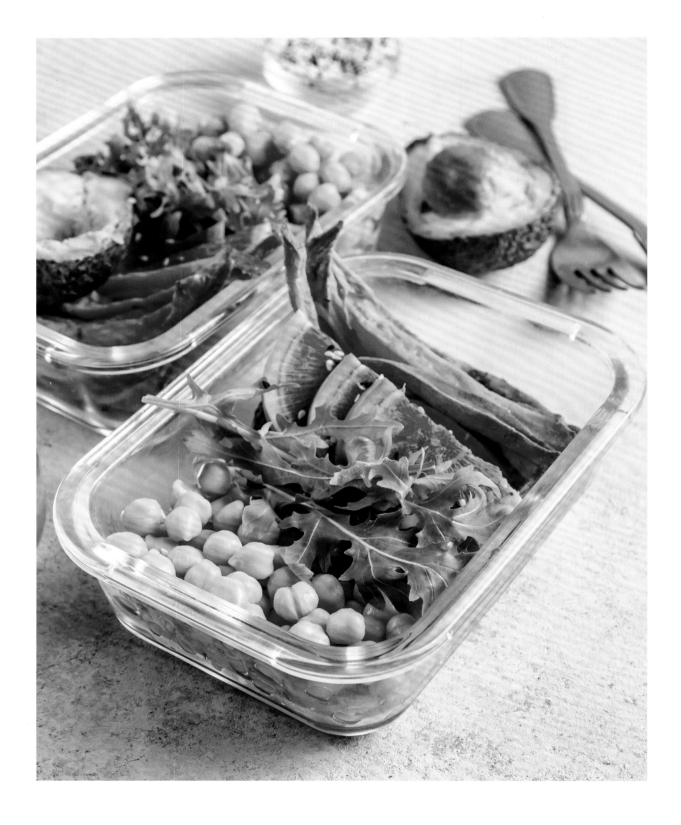

**MACRO-FOCUSED EATING =
HOLISTIC SUSTENANCE**

Holistic sustenance is achieved through cumulative nutrition. As you transition into a macro eating plan, spend time reflecting on where shifts are starting to occur in terms of mood, hunger, productivity, and motivation to exercise. Give yourself time to get used to a new way of understanding your nutritional needs. What you eat for lunch today, or even for a whole week, is not enough to completely alter the trajectory of the wellness path you're on. So commit to aligning food and lifestyle choices to positively impact your health as a whole while you get more familiar with tracking macros. Ask yourself:

- What do I need to do to have time to daily track my macros and exercise?
- How does my body feel after each meal or snack compared to how it used to?
- Am I more tired, bloated, and/or anxious after eating certain foods?
- Do I look forward to doing meal prep? Or does it feel like a massive chore? (If you answer "yes" to the latter, think about enlisting the help of a friend, partner, or family member to be your sous chef. Or, if you've got a bit of expendable income, outsource the task altogether via a delivery service that will customize macro meals for you.)
- What are you gaining in your life now that "what to eat" is becoming less of a stressor? Don't be surprised if free time, joy, body confidence, and other perks begin cropping up.

You will know your nutritional intake is providing sufficient fuel when you notice a distinct increase in physical energy, mental space, self-acceptance, and an ongoing desire to stay consistent with the changes you've made.

CULTIVATE A SUCCESS SQUAD

The first person on your wellbeing success team is you. Celebrating your progress should be a BIG self-care priority. But there will be times when external encouragement can help steer you through the challenges of making life changes. Do not rely on folks who try to debunk macro nutrition or devalue the adaptations you are making in eating habits. Release the negativity of these interactions by simply disengaging. Then go find some ease by sharing with supportive individuals equally interested in discovering heath-forward paths. Tell yourself "You got this!" daily. And on days when the mantra isn't sticking, phone or text a trusted confidante who is happy to be the bullhorn as many times as you need to hear it.

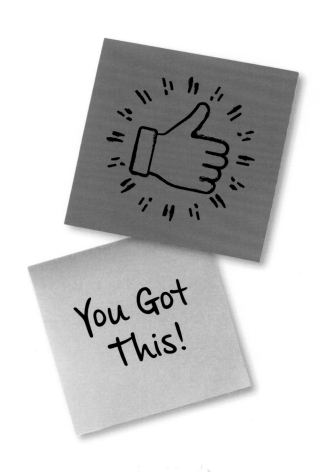

TERMINOLOGY CHEAT SHEET

As you dive deeper into crafting IIFYM menus, you will likely encounter a few of the following terms. It's also just a good idea to periodically refresh your knowledge of macro-related jargon (especially if you're the type of home cook who will be searching online for new recipes after sampling each one in this book).

- **Calorie deficit:** The body utilizing more calories than the amount gotten from foods eaten.
- **Simple carbs:** Carbohydrates that are digested easily so are able to provide short bursts of energy but are also more readily converted into fat (examples: white bread, table sugar, candy, chocolate, soda, corn syrup, fruit juice, and honey).
- **Complex carbs:** These carbohydrates take more time to digest, thanks to their fiber content. This also means we typically feel fuller for longer after eating—making them a more stable energy source than white rice, sugary drinks, or desserts. (Examples of complex carbs include multi-grain bread, oatmeal, brown rice, sweet potatoes, and whole-grain pasta.)
- **Carb tolerance:** Your body's metabolic and digestive response after carbohydrates have been eaten. This differs from gluten intolerance or glucose tolerance because it is not typically used to determine the risk of developing heart disease or diabetes. But it can be an early indicator that one has a gluten sensitivity or other food allergies.

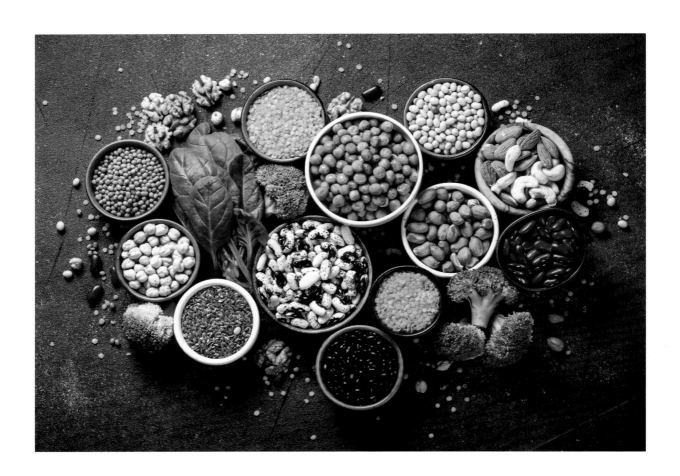

- **Animal protein:** Any protein source that originates from an animal. Many are considered *complete proteins*, but the trade-off, if over-consumed, is an increased risk of developing chronic cardiovascular issues and certain types of cancer. (Examples of animal proteins include eggs, cheese, whey, milk, red meat, poultry, fish.)
- **Plant protein:** Any protein source that originates from a plant. Plant protein can easily account for at least half of the protein you eat in a day, even if you're not vegetarian. (Examples of plant proteins include beans, peas, lentils, nuts, seeds, avocados, and some whole grains like quinoa, *teff*, *kamut*, and *farro*.)
- **Flexible dieting:** An approach to eating that is much less restrictive than many diets since there are no "forbidden" foods. Instead, the focus is on being strategic about when, in addition to how much, calorie-dense foods are consumed. Pizza, burgers, and milkshakes are all acceptable options in moderation (assuming macro amounts are properly being tracked daily).
- **Micronutrients:** Additional substances obtained from food that support essential processes within the human body. Vitamins, minerals, amino acids, fatty acids (omega-3 and omega-6), and antioxidants are all micronutrients.

Complete protein: A protein that provides all nine essential amino acids. Eggs, fish, milk, poultry, red meat, cheese, quinoa, buckwheat, and soy are complete proteins.

Farro: An ancient grain often used in Mediterranean-inspired meals that is high in fiber and protein; do not use if adhering to a gluten-free diet because it is a type of wheat.

Kamut: An ancient grain that works well as a substitute for whole wheat flour in bread baking or to thicken sauces. It is high in fiber, protein, iron, B vitamins, and manganese; it is also a type of wheat that should be avoided by those with a gluten-sensitivity or allergy.

Teff: An ancient grain frequently used in Ethiopian cooking that is a millet rather than type of wheat. This makes it a nutrient-dense, gluten-free alternative to use in bread, stuffing, or porridge recipes.

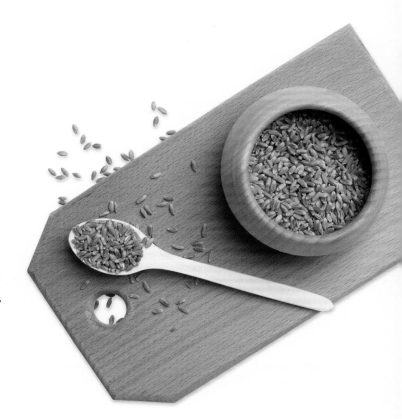

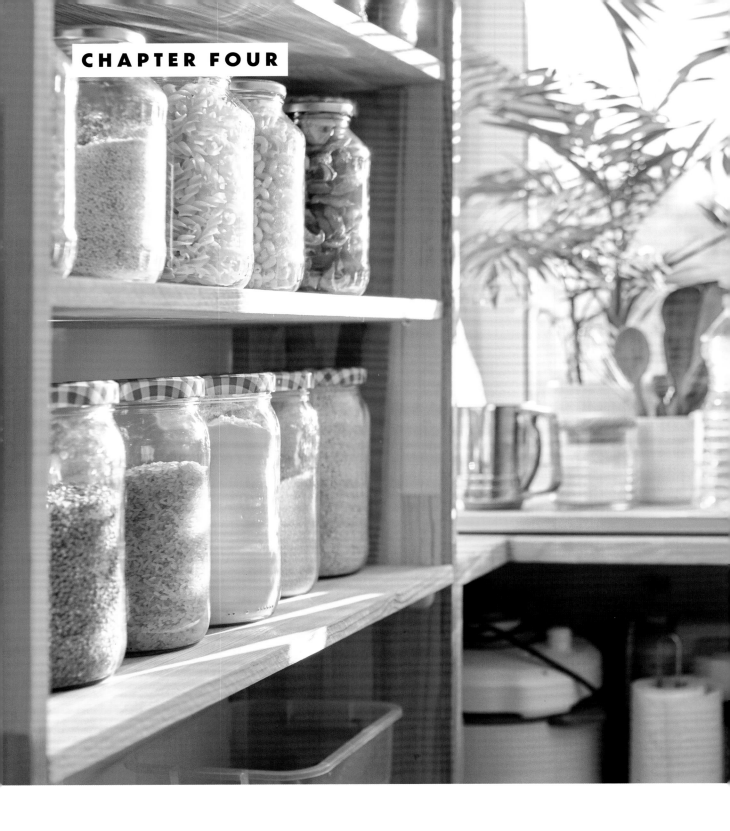

CHAPTER FOUR

MACRO COOKING MADE SIMPLER

Got a handle on how to crunch your macro numbers? Superb! Now it's time to join me in the kitchen. In this chapter, you'll find my top frugal foodies tips and buys, in addition to affordable allergy substitutions that won't break the bank.

I also share ideas about how to put my fave pantry staples to use. Although many of the flavor combos in the recipes I've created are delish, my hope is you'll embrace all the lifestyle and cooking ideas that follow as suggestions. Because the ability to "mix 'n' match" foods and tools to suit your needs is what macro eating is all about. I'm providing you with a culinary road map—not a homework assignment.

MACRO-FORWARD KITCHEN: 15 STAPLE INGREDIENTS

Any time of year, no matter the season—or the balance in my checking account—these are the basics I have in my cupboards. Having these items in steady supply allows me to meal prep whenever a break in my schedule permits rather than having to wait until the weekend or the next grocery delivery. However, what's a staple for me might not align with your dietary preferences or priorities. Harnessing an IIFYM perspective in your kitchen means you don't need special foods to reach your goals. So feel free to continue to use much of what you already have on hand to make nutritious meals while also trying a few of the staples from this list.

Rice

Choose your own adventure when selecting which type of rice becomes your default. I usually have a least two different kinds in my kitchen, which allows me to be flexible when meal prepping since rice is a suitable addition to breakfast bowls, lunch wraps, stir-fries, and much more. Be open to experimenting with brown, black, and wild rice since all three are high in fiber and antioxidants.

Legumes

If you're looking to diversify your protein sources, experimenting with different kinds of legumes is a good place to start. Another bonus of cooking with beans, lentils, and peas is that the majority are relatively inexpensive. Black beans and chickpeas (garbanzo beans) are always on standby in my cupboard since I frequently use both to level up soups, stews, and salads from a mere side to a main entrée in terms of satiety. My preference is to soak dry beans then cook a big batch—which I'll freeze to use as needed. But if my "backstock" is depleted or I am pressed for time, canned legumes work great too. For the recipes in this book where I call for a certain amount of beans, I am calling for beans that are already cooked; you may certainly substitute one 15-ounce (425 g) can for every 1½ to 2 cups (10 to 13 ounces [280 to 365 g]) of cooked beans. Just be sure to drain and rinse them before adding to any dish. Also, wait to salt the dish until the cook time is complete if the beans are not low sodium; salt to taste before serving instead.

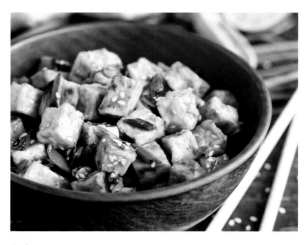

Tofu

Whereas some omnivores don't get the fanfare about these "curdled soymilk blocks," the proof lies in tofu being a sure bet for nailing protein needs. On average, a single cup of tofu has 20 grams of protein and no cholesterol; it's also a good source of digestible iron, calcium, zinc, and other minerals. Tofu types range from silken to extra-firm, which aren't always interchangeable, so be sure to follow the recipe. If this is your first foray into tofu, try Faux Fried Tofu on page 69.

Frozen Fruit

Smoothies and protein shakes will be a cinch, even if you only have a single bag of fruit in the freezer, but I recommend keeping bananas, peaches, and strawberries as your "go to" staples. This will allow you to mix up the flavor combinations to concoct a different version almost daily for a consecutive week. Another stellar use for frozen fruit is as an add-in to crumbles, bars, and other baked goods. Plus, a half cup of frozen berries on top of yogurt is a divine sweet treat that takes 3 minutes or less to assemble.

Local Produce

Farmer's markets are a macro connoisseur's best friend. The fresher the produce, the better. Eating in season means the veggies and fruits you're consuming have the highest nutrient content (with the least environmental impact). We all rely on imported, frozen, and canned versions at times. But there's no comparison in terms of nutrient density and flavor than produce sourced via farm-to-table methods. It's like saying a box of conventional, store-bought spaghetti is on par with from-scratch, hand-stretched noodles at an intimate bistro in Naples. Both are, of course, edible. However, there's a distinct difference when it comes to *quality*—and taste.

Oats

A low-cost, complex carb that is typically gluten-free, oats are a home cook's lifeline for feeding just about anyone on short notice. Consistently stocking 1 to 2 pounds of rolled oats gives you the ability to whip up oatmeal, granola, cookies, and crumbles like Breakfast Cobbler Cups on page 59. (If anyone in your household has a gluten allergy or gluten sensitivity, always check the packaging, as some oats are processed at a facility that also processes gluten-containing products.)

Lemons/Limes

My cooking routinely takes a hit whenever I forget to grab these citrus all-stars at the grocery store.

The hype behind balancing the "salt, acid, fat, and heat" proportions in recipes—popularized by celebrity chef Samin Nosrat—is actually warranted. If this concept is relatively new to you, try squeezing a quarter of a fresh lime or lemon onto a BBQ- or a chipotle-flavored entrée. You will likely notice how the spices suddenly "pop more." Adding citrus notes (acid) often increases the overall piquancy of a dish; it's what makes eats like Loaded Sweet Potato Salsa on page 101 such crowd pleasers.

Oil

If budget allows, give yourself permission to splurge on an array of oils, especially since a little goes a long way. Extra virgin olive oil, sesame seed, and tea seed oil (a neutral-flavored oil that is often used in Asian-inspired dishes) are three that are versatile for cooking savory food. The latter, in particular, contains a higher level of omega-3s than olive oil and can withstand extremely high cooking temps (up to 486°F [252°C])—so if you're a raw food fan or a grilling enthusiast, add it to your "must try" list. And coconut oil works well as a substitute for butter in many baking recipes.

Vinegar

Pick a kind, any kind. I am partial to rice vinegar and balsamic, but seriously, the most important thing is to be sure there's always a spare bottle tucked away. It's a quick remedy when you're out of salad dressing, or it's a solid base ingredient for numerous homemade condiments. A splash of red wine vinegar mixed with oil will add a bit of zest to freshly cut veggies. And apple cider vinegar is both cheap and versatile in terms of potential uses.

Vegetable Broth

Yes, it *is* quite simple to prepare a sizeable portion of veggie stock to freeze for use as needed, but until it is no longer possible to snag a 32-ounce (1.1 L) container for less than $3, I will continue to toss a couple cartons into my cart during every grocery run. Because using broth to add a bit of moisture to stir-fry or slow-roasting savory food

THE '411' ON OILS

Oils are a solid choice for hitting your daily macro plan's fat ratio. There are obviously *a lot* of options, so make selections based on nutritional specs and intended use such as:

Best picks for low to medium heat:
- Olive oil
- Unrefined coconut oil

Best picks for high heat:
- Refined coconut oil
- Grapeseed oil
- Peanut oil
- Safflower oil

Best picks for "flavor enhancement" (dressings and other condiments):
- Sesame oil
- Extra virgin olive oil

Best to leave on the shelf (due to lack of nutrients):
- Vegetable oil
- Shortening (of any kind)
- Canola oil

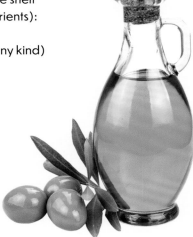

in the oven is a much better alternative than dribbling water into the pan—or dousing it with more oil. (If you're keeping a close eye on sodium intake, buy low-sodium stock and cut any salt in recipes at least by half, or omit altogether.)

Dairy-Free Milk

Stretching my money as far as I can is always a priority. We never seem to use an entire gallon of skim milk before it goes bad—even with a growing tween in the house! Food waste is one of my biggest pet peeves, so the much longer shelf life of plant-based milks is now the major draw for me in terms of choosing what to buy. These days, oat milk is my first choice, and I am always grateful there's a carton stashed away when I decide an hour before bedtime to prep overnight oats or Pecan Peach Porridge (page 63). But if oat milk turns out to not be your jam, sample other options like hemp, pea, soy, macadamia, coconut, or rice as opportunities arise.

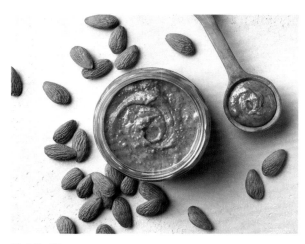

Nut Butter

Peanut butter may be a kid-friendly food, yet I have dozens of uses for it as well as for similar tasty varietals made of almonds, cashews, macadamia nuts, or hazelnuts. A dollop is usually my secret smoothie ingredient, as a flavor enhancement as well as to increase my protein intake. You'll certainly want to have some on hand to make Banana Maple Toast (page 67), Matcha Gems (page 123), or PB Boost (page 147). And if any household member is allergic to nuts, sunflower butter is a great alternative in terms of cost and shelf life.

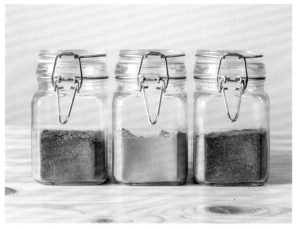

Spice Set

There's nothing worse than getting three-quarters of the way through a recipe and realizing you are missing one (or more) of the specified spices. If you routinely find that you're out of a spice, or you've made it this far with just salt and pepper, treat yourself to a set. Fresh spices add more pop to any dish—and they just taste better. To get the most out of any beginner bundle, be sure it has basil, cayenne, cilantro, cumin, dill, garlic, ginger, red pepper, rosemary, sage, thyme, and turmeric. (The other upshot to treating yourself to a set is that at least for a few months your spice shelf or drawer will look Marie Kondo–level organized to family and friends!)

Bread

Options for a macro *hit* breakfast or brunch abound if the bread box is not empty. Bread is not only allowed when tracking macros; it can actually provide a very versatile base for many meals. And, truly, any form will do—including gluten-free goods. Perhaps your household is forever fans of pita, naan, or the local bakery's baguettes. (Tortillas are in my fridge 24/7.) If you're still doubtful that bread can be part of a macro-based

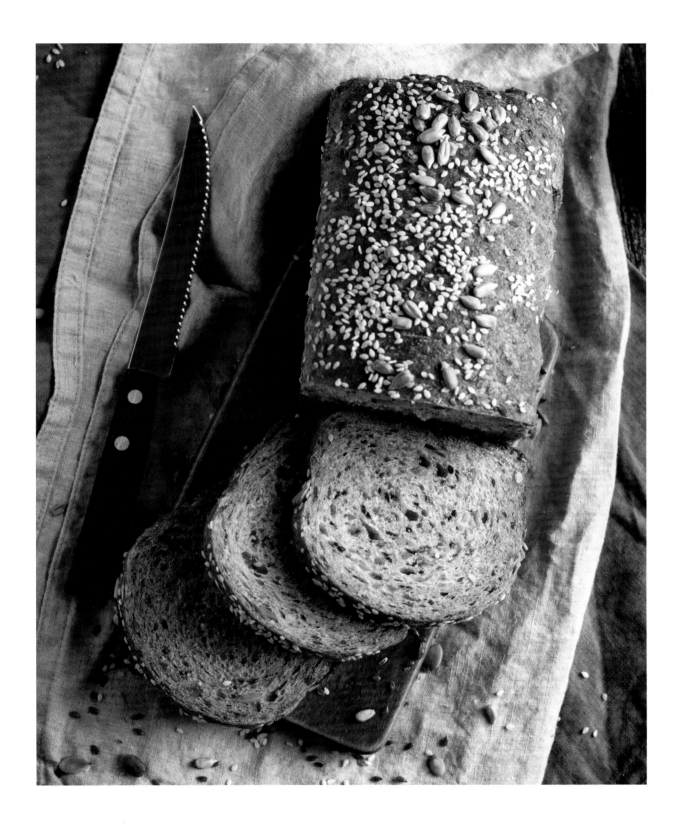

eating plan, test out the Avocado Stack (page 65), Banana Maple Toast (page 67), Black Bean Tostadas (page 93), Smoked Salmon Sliders (page 87), and BYO Brunch Burritos (page 57) as morning starters, especially if you're trying to bump up the protein ratio in your menu planning.

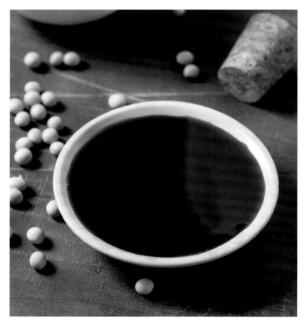

Tamari

Even if you don't have a gluten allergy, there's a strong probability you occasionally "break bread" with someone who does. Thus, spare yourself the headache of worry by swapping out that bottle of traditional soy sauce in your cupboard for this gluten-free alternative. Made from soybeans and no wheat, it's less salty than soy sauce but can be used in all the same ways. You could also try coconut aminos, another gluten-free condiment with a similar taste that is also soy free—and kosher. Either way, getting into the habit of utilizing a liquid seasoning instead of table or sea salt may help, over time, curb a tendency to oversalt food. Plus, if you enjoy Asian-inspired cuisine as much as I do, the majority of recipes you're likely to find will call for soy sauce or tamari.

MACRO-FORWARD KITCHEN: 7 ESSENTIAL KITCHEN TOOLS

This is not your mama's kitchen tools list. If you're over the age of 25, chances are you're already well stocked in terms of measuring cups, spatulas, knives, and an array of other basic home goods. So for those of us well seasoned at being the primary *chef-in-residence*, here's my "ride or die" list of equipment that has greatly improved my efficiency in the kitchen. While you will still be able to make the recipes in this book without these "essential" tools, they certainly make things simpler. As for me, no kitchen is complete without them.

High-Powered Blender

Let function be the deciding factor for which specific appliance in this category lands a coveted spot on your kitchen counter. I drink a smoothie a minimum of five times a week. I used to swear by a hand-held immersion blender for my food processing needs, but once I got a better-quality, high-speed blender, there was no going back. Any drink is ready in a minute or less; some blenders even heat up so much that they can make soup. So if your blender can process the ingredients in PB Boost (page 147) just as well as the veggies in the Carrot Ginger Bisque (page 103), then you're set!

Rice Cooker

I acquired my first rice cooker a few years ago, and it's been a complete game-changer ever since. Rice cookers can be used to perfectly cook most grains: quinoa, farro, millet, even a risotto that will come out as creamy as if it had simmered on the stove top. And over- (or under-) cooking whole grains can literally render dishes like Coconut Lemon Couscous (page 121) or Mixed Grain Salad (page 105) inedible. Due to its high-level of functionality, this is hands-down the one appliance I would instantly gift to everyone in my inner circle (if I had the disposable income to do so). Save yourself unnecessary stress by letting this appliance be your sous chef.

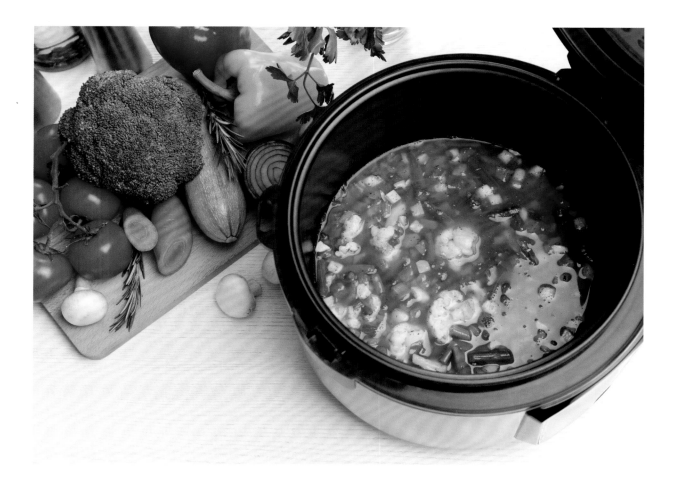

Slow Cooker or Multicooker (e.g., Instant Pot)

I was not an immediate multicooker convert. My slow cooker long held its coveted position in my cupboards. Even as a basic model that had cost less than $30, it had worked superb for almost a decade. However, the pandemic gifted me the inclination to test out a few new devices in the kitchen, including a multicooker. Now I equally adore them. It is not unusual for a single multicooker to make enough for dinner plus leftovers for two subsequent lunches. There is literally no easier way to make a meal in less than 30 minutes than using the multicooker—or several hours in the slow cooker if it's an entrée that can be left for hours unattended like Estofado Español (page 79) or Slow Cooker Meatballs (page 71).

Tofu Press

No matter how "firm" a block of tofu is labeled, it will be much easier to marinate, grill, fry, or bake if it's pressed for at least 15 to 20 minutes before cooking prep begins. Yes, stacking a few heavy books on top of two plates with a tofu block sandwiched between them is one pressing technique. But when you're short on time, that method isn't an effective option if trying to heat and eat a meal in less than a half hour. I also recommend the first press you purchase be low-maintenance in regard to cost, set-up, and sanitation; stick to stainless steel or dishwasher-safe plastic, upgrading to wood or bamboo if you're gradually less impressed by the starter version and find you use it often enough.

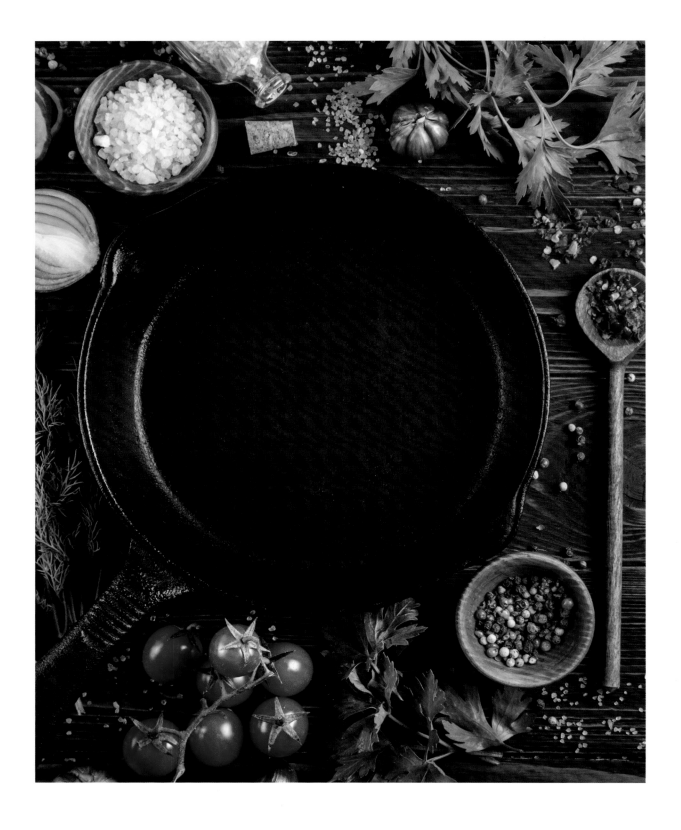

Pizza (or Baking) Stone

If there is one piece of kitchenware you are going to splurge on, this should be it. The one I currently own still looks impeccable after years of being put to use at various temperatures—and ovens—for flatbreads, pizzas, and calzones. You'll dually appreciate how evenly toasted the undersides of the Olive Focaccia (page 113) and Cheesy Eggplant Rounds (page 89) turn out if you do score a more high-end stone.

Cast Iron Pan or Pot

Everyone should own at least one cast iron cooking apparatus. Yes, it 100 percent does bring out flavors in food and will add a remarkable depth to your cooking skills. But the biggest contemporary selling point might just be the aesthetic. Any dish served up in one at a dinner party or holiday function instantly looks better. (Flip to the Crispy Fish Curry on page 83 for a prime example.)

Baking/Casserole Dishes with Lids

When you're starting any new way of eating, and particularly when following a macro approach, meal prepping can be your friend and help keep you on track. Being able to store prepared dishes that you can place right in the oven is a glorious feeling on busy weeknights when you need every task to go as efficiently as possible. Casserole sets can also eliminate the crazed search for matching pieces of plastic containers when there are leftovers you want to quickly pop back into the fridge before bed. Or for when you need a "no fuss" way to transport side dishes or desserts like Oven-Baked Apples and Kale (page 109) or Pumpkin Oat Bars (page 131) to work potlucks or holiday gatherings.

BONUS PRO TIP: SUSTAINABLE CLEANING MATERIALS

If you're taking the time to invest in quality equipment, do yourself a favor by swapping out old sponges and rags for eco-friendly successors. Reusable paper towels and cloths are made out of natural cotton and/or bamboo—and many are biodegradable. Also expect them to be nonabrasive, yet surprisingly quite effective at removing stains and smudges. In particular, I enjoy being able to toss them in the laundry with a load of towels (some can even go in the dishwasher), then simply air dry.

ALLERGEN-FRIENDLY MACRO COOKING

Modifying meals to meet multiple dietary needs in one household can feel like a perpetual struggle. Even for those living solo, having to come up with substitutions for familiar recipes to better suit your current nutritional goals may take more time than you can spare on a daily basis. The five swaps below are simple to execute; plus, they'll help you not surpass your target macros—without sacrificing taste in the process.

1. When you need to thicken a sauce or make gravy, while also keeping it gluten-free, use ½ tablespoon arrowroot powder, cornstarch, or rice or potato flour in place of 1 tablespoon wheat flour.
2. Mixing equal parts miso paste and tahini, then combining with a splash of water and a dash of rice vinegar, creates a dairy- and gluten-free salad dressing or dip. The base flavor can be easily altered by adding garlic, ginger, and/or mustard when you're in the mood for a bit of variety.
3. Tofu blended with lemon juice is a low-fat and dairy-free alternative to sour cream. And if a recipe needs to be dairy-free and calls for heavy cream, use canned coconut milk (well stirred).
4. If you're missing having a breakfast sweet on weekend mornings, apple butter on gluten-free toast is an option that's more affordable—and less caloric—than most pastries.
5. Seaweed, coconut aminos, or oyster sauce are suitable replacements for fish sauce in many recipes if there's a seafood allergy in your household.

By design, the recipes I've created for this book are suitable for various allergies and food preferences (see box below). However, it is still important to double-check ingredient labels, whether it's premade sauces and premixed spices/seasonings, or something that is usually gluten free, like oats. For example, I always ensure the packaging on oats (and oat flour) explicitly states the product is gluten-free before buying. Even if "most kinds" of a certain product are

LOOK FOR THESE ICONS AT THE TOP OF EACH RECIPE PAGE:

 indicates the recipe is vegetarian (or there's a vegetarian option)

 indicates the recipe is vegan (or there's a vegan option)

 indicates the recipe is dairy-free (or there's a dairy-free option)

 indicates the recipe is gluten-free (or there's a gluten-free option)

 indicates the recipe is nut-free (or there's a nut-free option)

 indicates the recipe is soy-free (or there's a soy-free option)

 indicates the recipe is a one-pot meal

usually free of a particular allergen, it is best to never assume if you're preparing meals for folks with medically diagnosed food allergies.

And if you find yourself needing a substitution that I haven't referenced or suggested, there's a plethora of allergen-friendly products now available in just about any market that you can swap in to still meet your target macros. Here's a list of common verbiage associated with allergenic foods to be on the lookout for when shopping:

- Gluten: Wheat in any form (flour, protein, starch, grass, oil, extract), durum, barley, malt, bulgur
- Dairy: whey, casein, sodium caseinate
- Eggs: albumen (albumin), mayonnaise, meringue, lecithin, lysozyme
- Seafood: fish sauce, fish stock, crevette, caviar, prawn, roe, any broth/powder/extract derived from shellfish
- Nuts: arachis (arachic/arachide) oil, goober peas/goobers, mandelonas (the "faux nut"), some nougats and marzipans
- Soy: bean curd (yuba), miso, natto, soya flour, tempeh, tamari, textured vegetable protein (TVP), edamame, kinnoko flour, shoyu sauce, soy lecithin

Allergen Apps: Download one of these apps to reference while grocery shopping, dining out, or traveling to stay in the know about the latest allergen-friendly options.
- Spoonful
- Fig
- Yuka
- Soosee
- Spokin

Food allergy: A food allergy occurs when the body's immune system is triggered to perceive specific foods as a threat. Often, ingesting even a small amount of the allergen can cause digestive problems, rash, hives, or breathing issues. The eight most common food allergens are milk, eggs, fish, shellfish, tree nuts, peanuts, wheat, and soy.

Food sensitivity: Food sensitivities are also referred to as *food intolerance* because it is diagnosed when one's digestive system is unable to process particular food(s). This usually results in bloating, gas, diarrhea, and/or abdominal pain. Unlike a food allergy, however, food sensitivities are not life-threatening.

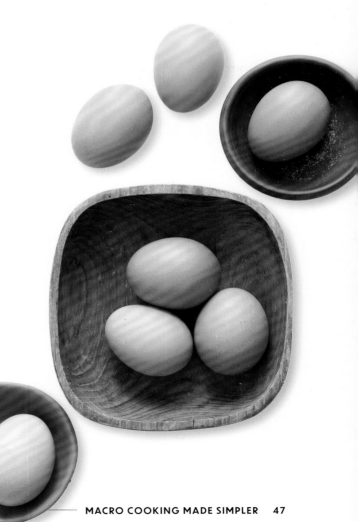

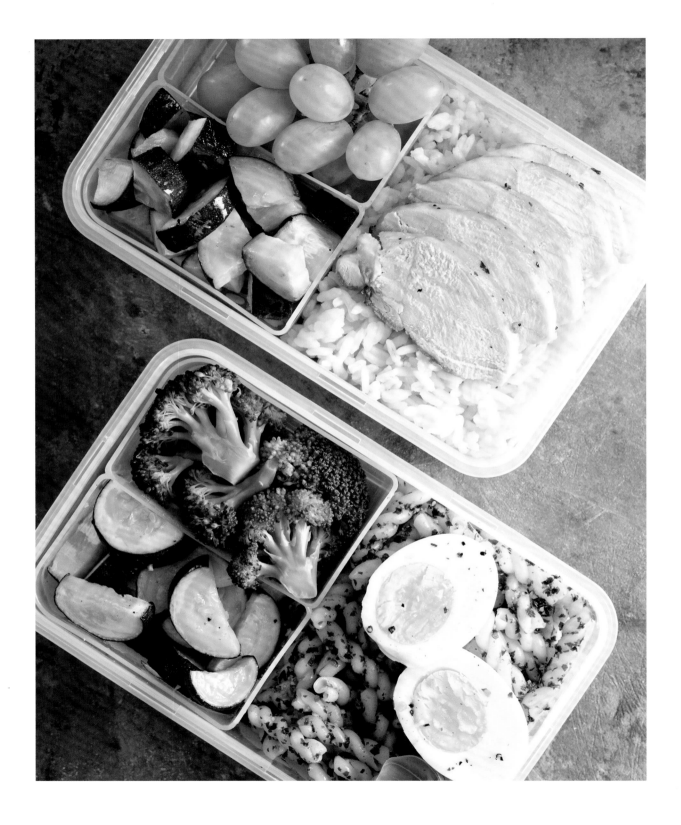

FRUGAL FOODIE TIPS

Feel like you need a guide to macro cooking on a budget? You've got one right here! I created the following recipes for breakfasts, mains, sides, snacks, and beverages keeping in mind ingredients you likely already have at home—or that won't put a noticeable dent in your bank account. Here are a few additional money-saving ideas:

Cook in Batches

This time-saving tip is also one of the most effective ways to ensure macro meal prep stays affordable. For example, here are some prime pairings from this book that will add up to cost savings if made in the same week by utilizing similar ingredients: Cinnamon Batatas (page 137) and Loaded Sweet Potato Salsa (page 101); BYO Brunch Burritos (page 57) and Black Bean Tostadas (page 93); Honey Walnut Chicken (page 91) and Cilantro Lime Chicken Salad (page 95). For other pairings and to create your own, see page 50.

Peruse Bulk Options

The emphasis here is on *browsing* as you become accustomed to buying larger (or smaller) quantities when it makes the most sense. Because of how much recipe testing I do, it's not unusual for me to pop into our local food co-op to pick up small amounts of dried spices as needed instead of purchasing whole jars that will likely expire before they're even halfway empty. I reserve purchasing in mass quantities for staples I am guaranteed to use multiple times a week, like rice, tofu, peanut butter, and frozen fruit.

Shop Less

Schedule when you'll go to the grocery store...like an appointment. Scaling back unnecessary trips to the store means you're less likely to come home with items you're trying to limit consumption of.

And a decrease in *impulse buys* has the added benefit of saving you money by preventing you from stuffing the fridge with items bought "on sale," yet will likely be tossed later, barely used.

Embrace a DIY Mentality

Make as many things from scratch as time and your sanity will allow. For example, you can get three to four times the amount of beans if you purchase dried versus canned. Same goes for allergen-friendly desserts, sauces, dressings, and condiments.

Repurpose Leftovers

Yesterday's sweet potato soup is a tasty nondairy base for a black bean and avocado quesadilla. And just about any combo of veggies can be used to create a new soup by simply simmering in veggie broth for 20 minutes.

Notice Expiration Dates

One of the simplest ways to avoid food waste is to check the "best by" dates of perishable items. Items like cheese, bread, flour, fruit, and veggies can be frozen if transferred to airtight containers or resealable plastic bags before they start to spoil. Also prioritize buying produce with a longer shelf life such as apples, pears, broccoli, and cabbage.

Use Tech Tools

Once you have tried the 50 recipes in this book, look no further than Pinterest and Instagram for additional inspiration. Give yourself permission to experiment with making low-cost versions of any dishes or snacks that align with your target macros. And don't forget the tracking apps listed on page 31. Some can merge your grocery and recipe lists better than a paid assistant IRL.

MEAL PREP PLANNER

These recipes require several of the same ingredients, so set yourself up for success, plus maximize time spent in the kitchen by prepping these dishes together at the beginning of the week. Feel free to pair with others you're already seasoned at making too. Mix and match the optional ingredients for each dish to keep your culinary creativity flowing, while staying within a manageable macro range.

Use this space to write down staple ingredients you always have on hand or ingredients for recipes you have in frequent rotation.

_____

_____

_____

_____

_____

_____

_____

_____

_____

_____

_____

_____

_____

_____

_____

_____

_____

_____

WEEK 1
TARGET MACROS
Mixed Grain Salad, Sesame Farro, Cajun "Hot Hash"
Others:

WEEK 2
TARGET MACROS
Protein Power Pancakes, Pumpkin Oat Bars, PB Boost
Others:

WEEK 3
TARGET MACROS
Carrot Ginger Bisque, Gajar Halwa, The Ultimate DIY Bowl
Others:

WEEK 4
TARGET MACROS
Honey Walnut Chicken, Cilantro Lime Chicken, Cucumber Rolls
Others:

WEEK 7
TARGET MACROS
Harvest Rice, Zucchini Arancini, Tex-Mex Stuffed Squash
Others:

WEEK 5
TARGET MACROS
Breakfast Cobbler Cups, Pecan Peach Porridge, Pumpkin Oat Bars
Others:

WEEK 8
TARGET MACROS
BYO Brunch Burritos, Black Bean Tostadas, Avocado Stack
Others:

WEEK 6
TARGET MACROS
Faux Fried Tofu, TLT Boats, Avocado Stack
Others:

WEEK 9
TARGET MACROS
Loaded Sweet Potato Salsa, Cinnamon Batatas, Caribbean Jambalaya
Others:

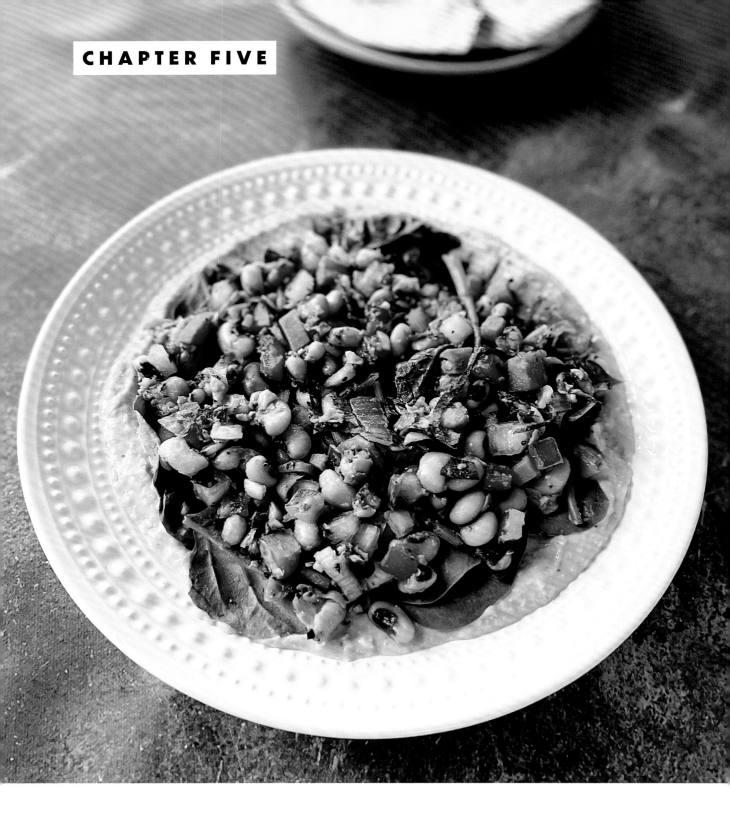

CHAPTER FIVE

MACRO RECIPES
MADE DELICIOUS

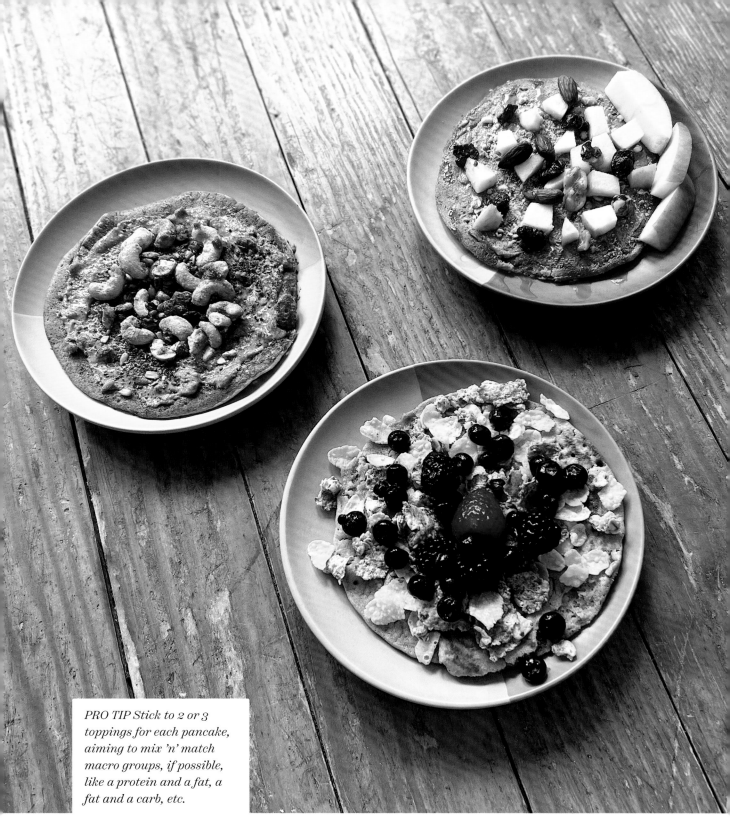

PRO TIP Stick to 2 or 3 toppings for each pancake, aiming to mix 'n' match macro groups, if possible, like a protein and a fat, a fat and a carb, etc.

PROTEIN POWER PANCAKES

What I adore about this pancake recipe is the base batter works with a wide variety of toppings, providing a valid excuse to use hazelnut spread and maple syrup during the same meal. Another highlight is one stack usually keeps me well-fueled until about midday, thanks to the protein powder, so this is an excellent breakfast choice when your day's schedule seems particularly packed.

Ingredients

¾ cup (92 g) whole wheat flour

¾ cup (92 g) oat flour

½ cup (125 g) protein powder

1 tablespoon (14 g) baking powder

1 to 2 teaspoons ground nutmeg or cloves

Pinch of salt

1 cup (235 ml) milk of choice

½ cup (128 g) applesauce

¼ cup (60 ml) coconut oil

OPTIONAL TOPPINGS

1 cup (150 g) fresh berries or chopped fruit

1 cup (250 g) nut butter

½ cup (70 g) granola, cereal, or nuts

¼ cup (74 g) hazelnut spread

¼ cup (85 g) honey or (60 ml) maple syrup

Directions

1. In a large bowl, mix the flours, protein powder, baking powder, and spices. Stir in the milk and applesauce until well combined (no dry spots).

2. Grease a small skillet set over medium heat with a small amount of coconut oil (a little goes a long way). Pour in the pancake batter for each pancake.

3. As soon as bubbles start to appear on the tops of the pancakes, about 3 minutes, flip them over. Cook until the second side has browned. Remove from the skillet and repeat with the remaining oil and batter.

4. Mix and match optional toppings once plated.

YIELD 4 servings

PER SERVING 337 calories; 23 g fat; 7 g protein; 43 g carbohydrate

PREP TIME 10 mins **TOTAL TIME** 25 mins

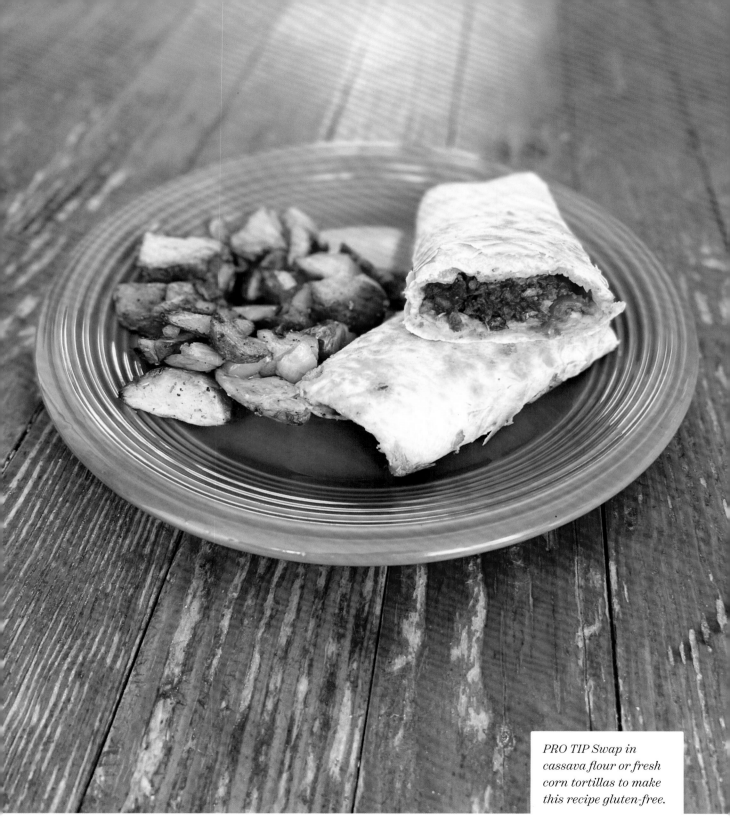

PRO TIP Swap in cassava flour or fresh corn tortillas to make this recipe gluten-free.

BYO BRUNCH BURRITOS

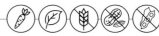

Brunch is absolutely in the top five of my simple pleasures list. (Especially on the weekend!) And I have gotten so good at mastering the "crunch" technique for stand-out burritos, I rarely order one at restaurants anymore. The trick is to essentially fuse the egg and tortilla together in the skillet so that the burrito can be rolled up in the skillet, toasting both the core and the outside. The result: edible perfection in terms of taste and speedy cook time. Serve them with a side of potatoes for a perfect brunch meal.

Ingredients

2 tablespoons (30 ml) olive oil

2 large eggs (or ½ cup [120 ml] egg substitute)

2 large flour tortillas (see Pro Tip)

2 cups (56 g) fresh spinach

1 cup (250 g) crumbled or chopped chorizo (optional)

1 large bell pepper, chopped (optional)

½ cup (56 g) shredded Cheddar cheese (optional)

Pinch of salt

Pinch of black pepper

Directions

1. Add 1 tablespoon (15 ml) oil to a large skillet set over medium-low heat.

2. Crack 1 egg into a bowl and whisk before pouring into the skillet.

3. Immediately after the egg starts to bubble, place 1 tortilla on top of it and press down with a spatula.

4. Wait 4 to 5 minutes, then carefully lift a small part of the tortilla to check if the egg has begun to stick to it. Once it has, flip the tortilla and egg "shell" over.

5. Place half the spinach and half of the other toppings, as desired, on one side of the tortilla. Add a pinch of salt and pepper, then gently begin to roll using a spatula.

6. Once rolled, toast on each side until the outer layer of the tortilla gets crispy or slightly browned. Remove from the skillet and repeat with the remaining ingredients.

7. Cool slightly before cutting in half.

YIELD 2 servings

PER SERVING 641 calories; 25 g fat; 47 g protein; 54 g carbohydrate

PREP TIME 5 mins **TOTAL TIME** 20 mins

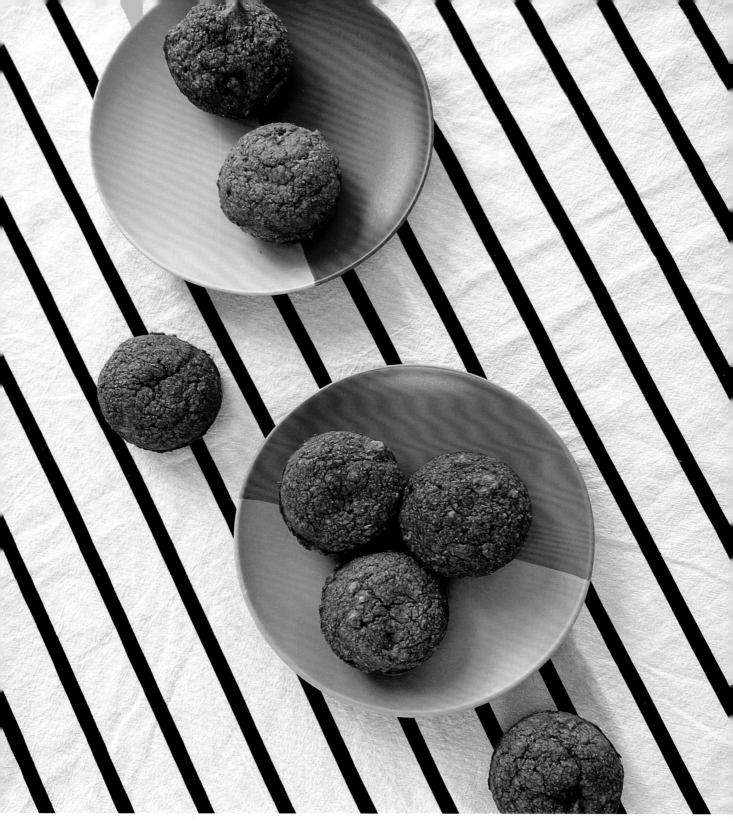

BREAKFAST COBBLER CUPS

Brekkie fare that can be assembled the night before will always have a front row seat in my recipe box. I usually make this particular one with apples, but feel free to swap in rhubarb, peaches, bananas, or pears, depending on what's in season where you live.

Ingredients

Nonstick cooking spray

½ cup (68 g) pastry flour or all-purpose flour

¾ cup (160 g) cane sugar or (180 ml) maple syrup

¼ cup (35 g) granola

¼ cup (60 ml) coconut oil, melted

¼ cup (64 g) nut butter

1 tablespoon (8 g) ground cinnamon

½ teaspoon salt

2 cups (about ½ lb [227 g]) cut-up fresh fruit (apples, peaches, etc., cut into chunks)

Directions

1. Preheat the oven to 350°F (180°C, or gas mark 4) and spray a muffin tray with nonstick cooking spray.

2. In a medium bowl, combine the flour, cane sugar, and granola with a fork or a pastry blender until small crumbs form.

3. In a separate medium bowl, stir together the coconut oil, nut butter, cinnamon, and salt. Add the fruit and toss to coat.

4. Combine the fruit mixture with the dry ingredients.

5. Spoon the batter into a muffin tin and bake until a toothpick inserted into the center of one comes out mostly clean, 25 to 30 minutes.

6. Cool a few minutes in the pan before removing the muffins to a wire rack to cool completely.

> *PRO TIP Store cups in an airtight container for up to three days in the fridge or two days at room temp. Reheat if desired in the microwave for 10 seconds.*

YIELD 12 cups (3 per serving)

PER SERVING 373 calories; 23 g fat; 5 g protein; 62 g carbohydrate

PREP TIME 15 mins **TOTAL TIME** 40 mins

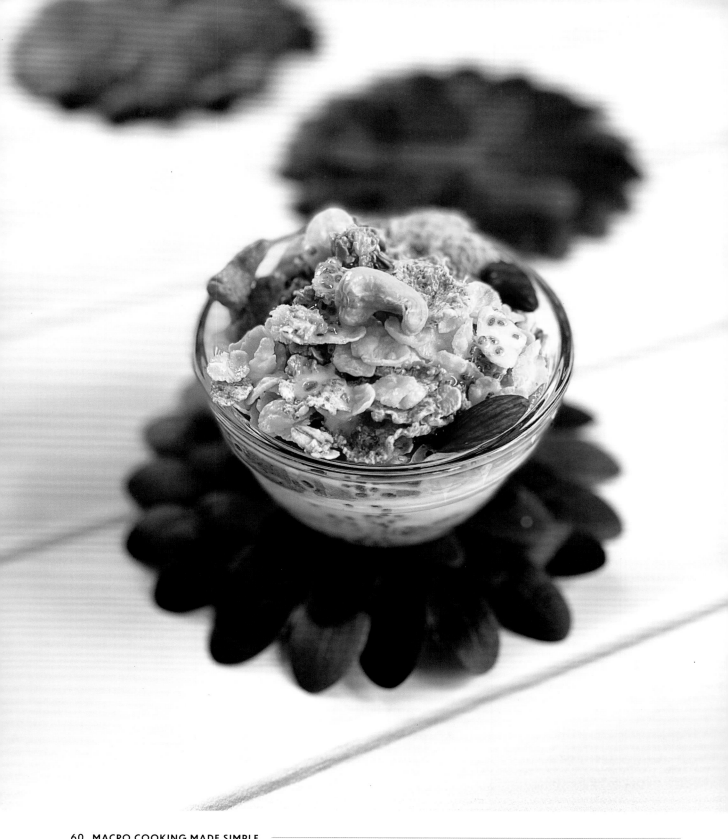

CHIA PARFAIT

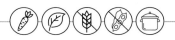

For the longest time, chia seeds held zero appeal to me. But a woman can only eat so much flaxseed, so I finally succumbed to giving chia a try. My only regret now is that I didn't do it sooner. Over time, like me, you may find it more versatile than flax when you need a fiber boost and a recipe without a bunch of additional steps...like this parfait.

Ingredients

1 cup (235 ml) whole or dairy-free milk

2 tablespoons (20 g) chia seeds

¼ cup (64 g) vanilla Greek or nondairy yogurt

1 tablespoon (16 g) nut butter

2 to 3 tablespoons (18 g) granola

2 teaspoons (10 g) chopped nuts or dried fruit

Directions

1. To make the chia pudding, combine the milk and chia seeds in a bowl. Cover and refrigerate for at least 45 minutes (but you can leave it for over an hour, or even overnight, if necessary).

2. When ready to serve, spoon the yogurt on top of the chia pudding. Then layer on the nut butter, granola, and nuts or fruit. Serve immediately.

YIELD 1 serving

PER SERVING 462 calories; 26 g fat; 23 g protein; 37 g carbohydrate

PREP TIME 5 mins **TOTAL TIME** 50 mins

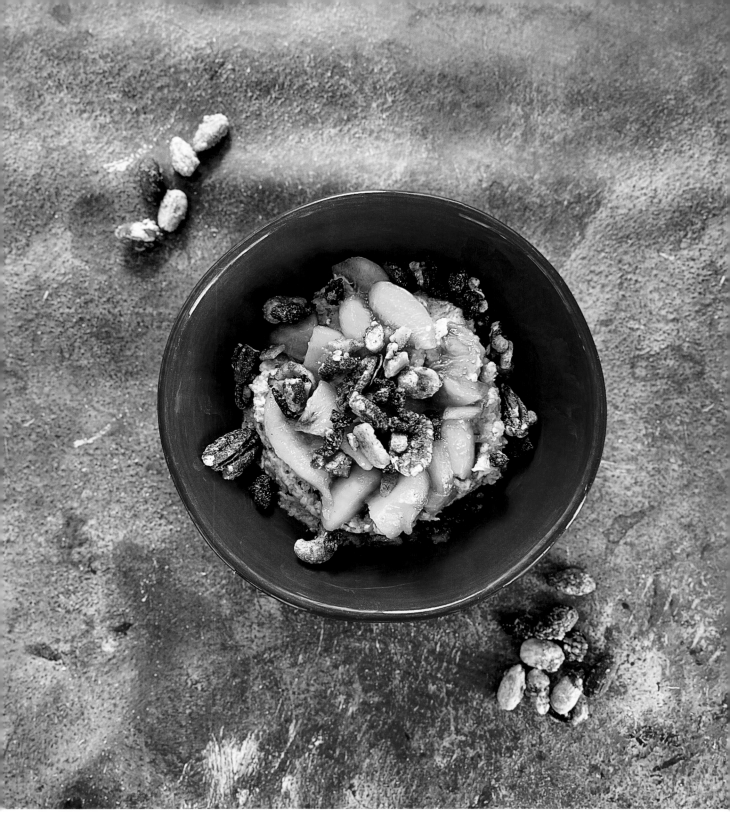

PECAN PEACH PORRIDGE

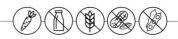

Peaches are a low-glycemic fruit, which means they have minimal effect on blood sugar. So if you're sensitive to sugar spikes and crashes, they're an ideal fruit to start your day with by adding them to cold cereals, smoothies, and warm breakfast nosh, like this porridge. But don't let the name fool you—it's also a quick, hearty, and comforting snack to whip together any time of day. (And though pecans add a nice crunch and some good fats, this porridge is equally delicious if you need to cut them out for dietary reasons.)

Ingredients

5 cups (1.2 L) whole milk or unsweetened vanilla nondairy milk

2 cups (160 g) rolled oats

½ teaspoon ground cinnamon

½ teaspoon salt

¾ cup (112 g) frozen sliced peaches

¼ cup (85 g) honey

2 tablespoons (31 g) pecans or dried fruit (optional)

Directions

1. In a medium saucepan over medium heat, combine the milk, oats, cinnamon, and salt then bring to a low boil.

2. Reduce the heat to low and continue to stir until the oats are tender, 5 to 10 minutes.

3. Meanwhile, in a second medium saucepan over low heat, cook the peaches and honey until the mixture has a syrup base and the peaches are warmed thoroughly, 4 to 5 minutes.

4. Divide the porridge among four bowls.

5. Scoop one-quarter of the cooked peaches into each bowl and top with pecans (if using) or dried fruit.

YIELD 4 servings

PER SERVING 498 calories; 10 g fat; 20 g protein; 83 g carbohydrate

PREP TIME 5 mins **TOTAL TIME** 15 mins

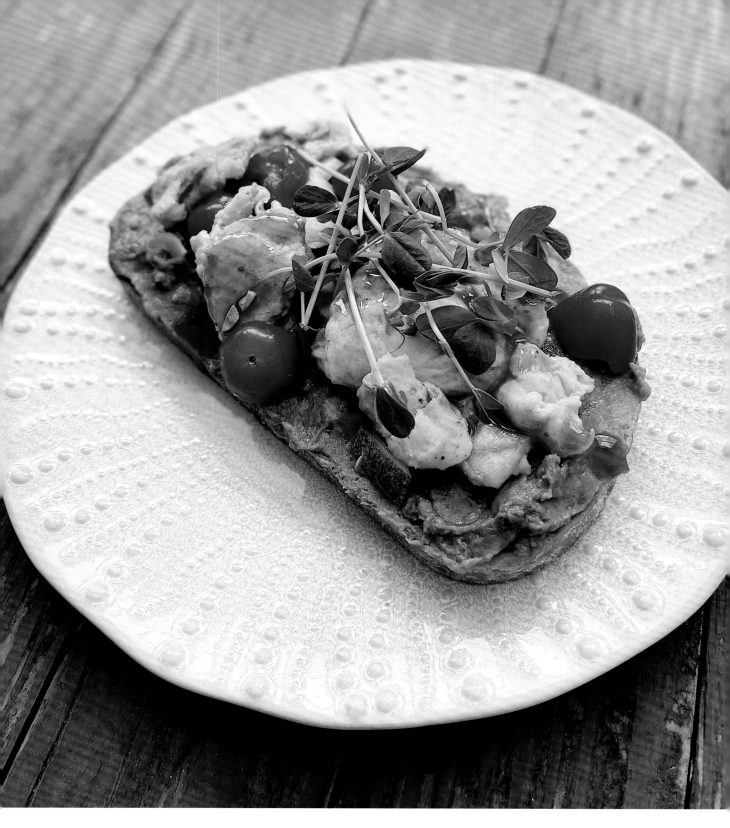

AVOCADO STACK

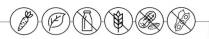

Another photographer recently mentioned that nearly every other food pic he sees of mine is of avocado toast. At first, I tried to deny it, then realized that was likely true...considering how often I make it at home and order it when dining out. Due to their being an excellent source of healthy fat, I am not remotely ashamed of being such an avo fangirl, and neither will you be after trying this toast. The flavor and texture combinations are so satisfying, you'll be tempted to consume two pieces in one sitting.

Ingredients

1 slice sourdough or gluten-free bread

½ large avocado

¼ teaspoon salt

1 medium or large egg (or equivalent egg substitute)

¼ cup (3 ounces [85 g]) sliced cherry tomatoes

2 to 3 teaspoons (8 g) diced onion (optional)

Pea shoots or other microgreens, for garnish

2 or 3 teaspoons (15 ml) sriracha sauce (optional)

Directions

1. Toast the bread.

2. Meanwhile, use a spoon to scoop out the inside of the avocado and transfer to a bowl. Mash it with a fork until smooth, mixing in half the salt while doing so. Set aside.

3. In a skillet, scramble or fry the egg to your liking.

4. Spread the avocado on top of the toast. Top with the egg, tomatoes, onion (if using), the remaining salt, and pea shoots and sriracha, if using.

> PRO TIP Pre-mashing the avocado makes it easier to spread, no matter the type of bread you're using and no matter how ripe the avocado is.

YIELD 1 serving

PER SERVING 373 calories; 22 g fat; 8 g protein; 36 g carbohydrate

PREP TIME 5 mins **TOTAL TIME** 10 mins

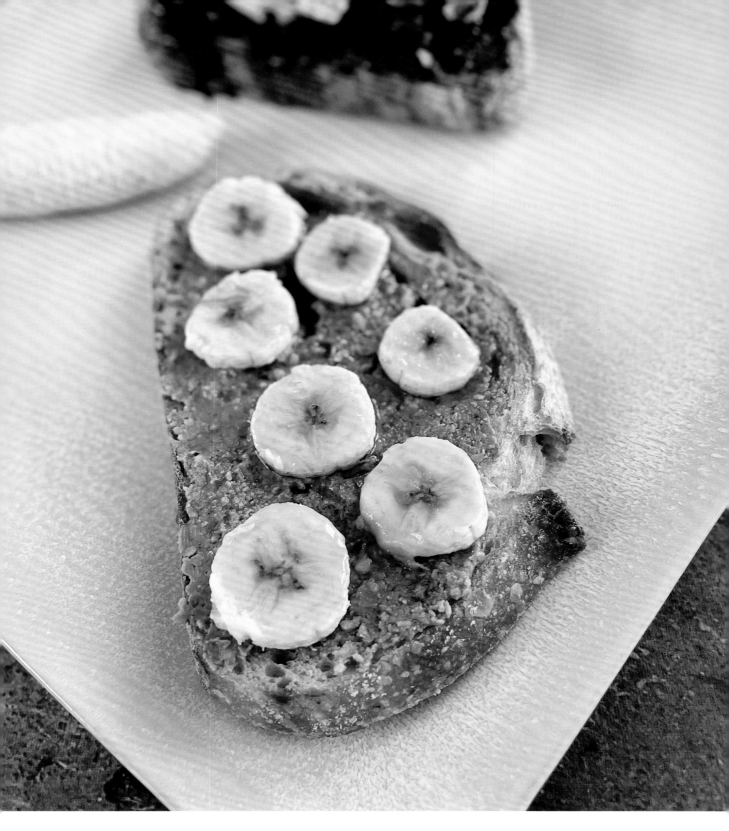

BANANA MAPLE TOAST

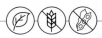

Texture *strongly* influences taste for me. I was one of those rare children who actually loathed peanut butter and jelly sandwiches. In hindsight, I think it was mainly because it would be more than a decade before I knew "crunchy" nut butters existed. (Maple syrup and agave also trump jam any day for me.) This toast is a quick option for brekkie when a proper nosh is a must after a morning workout before dashing off to the office or morning carpool. It's also an anytime snack that checks multiple "boxes" in terms of your ratios. Call me bougie all you want, but you got to admit this toastie is much more satisfying than the average PB&J.

Ingredients

1 slice sourdough or gluten-free bread

2 tablespoons (32 g) almond or peanut butter

½ small banana, sliced

1 tablespoon (15 ml) pure maple syrup

Salt (optional)

Directions

1. Toast the bread.

2. Spread the almond butter over the toast.

3. Top with the banana slices and drizzle with maple syrup.

4. Sprinkle with salt, if desired, before savoring that first bite.

> *PRO TIP Try slathering toast in hazelnut spread (topped with chopped nuts) as an alternate delish—and nutritious—"ready in a flash" breakfast option.*

YIELD 1 serving

PER SERVING 415 calories; 20 g fat; 7 g protein; 51 g carbohydrate

PREP TIME 5 mins **TOTAL TIME** 5 mins

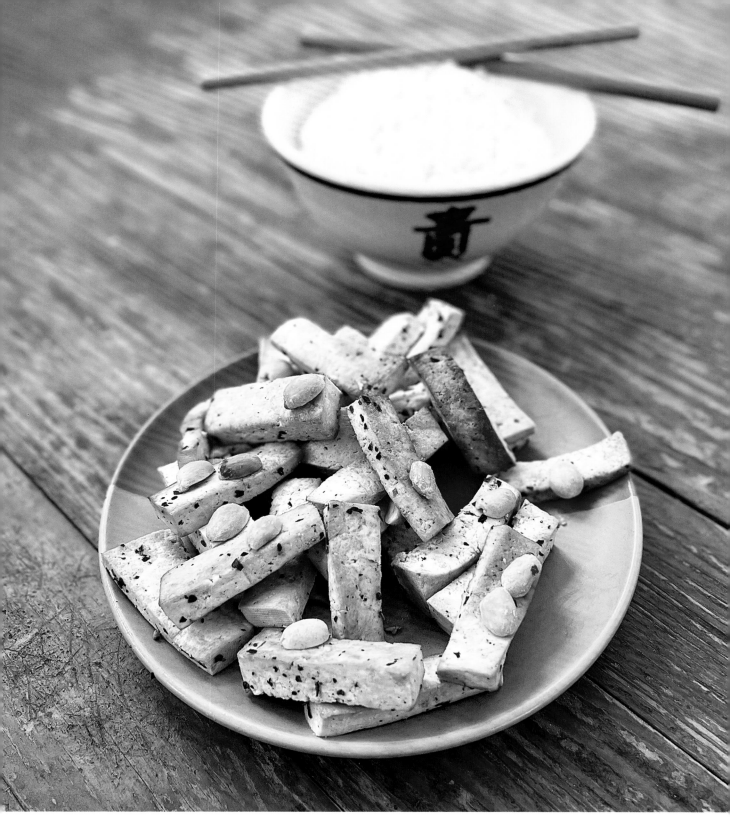

FAUX FRIED TOFU

Herein lies the one recipe I would stake my life is worth every millisecond spent prepping. I really had come to think it just wasn't within my culinary ability to produce the non-soggy tofu I get with takeout. But it turns out the secret lies in the quality and length of time the tofu is pressed. Which means don't cut corners on either—and you'll likely come to love this dish as much as I do. Serve it with cooked rice, cold soba noodles, or stir-fried vegetables.

Ingredients

1 package (14 ounces [396 g]) firm or extra-firm tofu, drained

2 tablespoons (30 ml) sesame oil

2 tablespoons (30 ml) soy sauce or tamari

1 teaspoon garlic powder

Black pepper, to taste

¼ to ½ cup (56 to 112 g) peanuts (optional)

Directions

1. Preheat the oven to 425°F (220°C, or gas mark 7).

2. Place the tofu inside a tofu press (or see Pro Tip) and press for at least 10 minutes—the longer the better!

3. Once pressed, slice the tofu into 1-inch strips.

4. Warm the sesame oil in an oven-safe medium skillet (cast iron is great) over medium heat. Add the tofu and cook, without moving, 1 to 2 minutes before adding the soy sauce, garlic powder, and black pepper.

5. Cook the tofu on all sides until it turns golden and begins to crisp, 5 to 7 minutes.

6. Transfer the skillet to the hot oven and bake until crispy, about 15 minutes.

7. Add peanuts as a final garnish before serving, if desired.

> PRO TIP If you don't have a tofu press, an alternate method for Step 2 is to wrap the whole block in an absorbent clean kitchen towel or a few layers of paper towel before placing it onto a plate. Top with another plate and place a heavy, sturdy item on top to press the tofu for 15 to 20 minutes. (I used to use my cast iron skillet for this before I owned a press.)

YIELD 4 servings

PER SERVING 153 calories; 12 g fat; 11 g protein; 3 g carbohydrate

PREP TIME 15 mins **TOTAL TIME** 35 mins

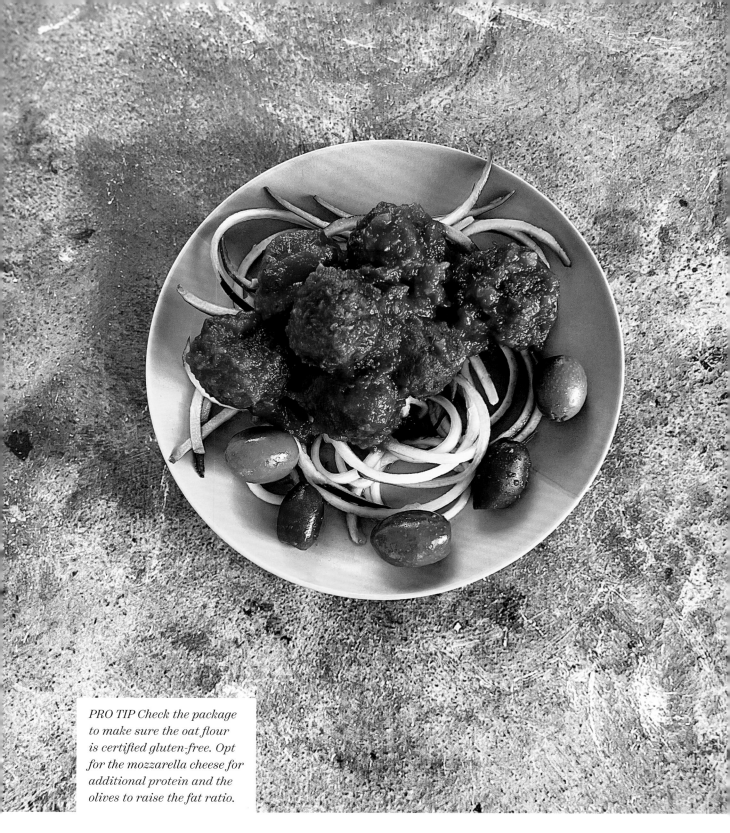

PRO TIP *Check the package to make sure the oat flour is certified gluten-free. Opt for the mozzarella cheese for additional protein and the olives to raise the fat ratio.*

SLOW COOKER MEATBALLS

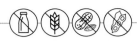

I love a meal that can be prepped the night before or first thing in the morning. It means one less task taking up mental space since I already know what we'll be eating for dinner. Also, any excuse to savor zoodles is a FTW move in my book; use them however you prefer—raw or lightly sautéed. But give yourself the option to sub in spaghetti (traditional or gluten-free) on days when a bump in carb intake is needed.

Ingredients

1½ pounds (680 g) ground turkey

½ cup (62 g) oat flour or bread crumbs

2 large eggs (or ½ cup [120 ml] egg substitute)

1 tablespoon (14 g) minced garlic

1 tablespoon (8 g) onion powder

1 tablespoon (4 g) dried oregano

1 tablespoon (8 g) salt

1 tablespoon (4 g) ground black pepper

Nonstick cooking spray

1 cup (250 g) prepared arrabbiata or marinara sauce, divided

¼ cup (60 ml) water

4 cups (12 ounces [340 g]) zucchini noodles ("zoodles")

1 cup (112 g) shredded mozzarella cheese (optional)

1 cup (250 g) pitted olives (optional)

Directions

1. In a large bowl, add the turkey, flour, eggs, garlic, and spices and mix with your hands until combined.

2. Form into 1- or 2-inch meatballs and set aside.

3. Lightly coat the bottom and sides of a slow cooker with the cooking spray, then add the meatballs. Add ¼ cup sauce and the water.

4. Cover and cook on LOW for 4 hours (or on HIGH for 2).

5. Pour the remaining sauce over the meatballs, replace the lid, and cook on LOW for an additional 30 to 45 minutes.

6. Serve over raw or lightly sautéed zoodles, topped with the cheese and/or olives, if desired.

YIELD 4 servings (4 or 5 meatballs each)

PER SERVING 356 calories; 8 g fat; 47 g protein; 25 g carbohydrate

PREP TIME 20 mins **TOTAL TIME** 5 hours

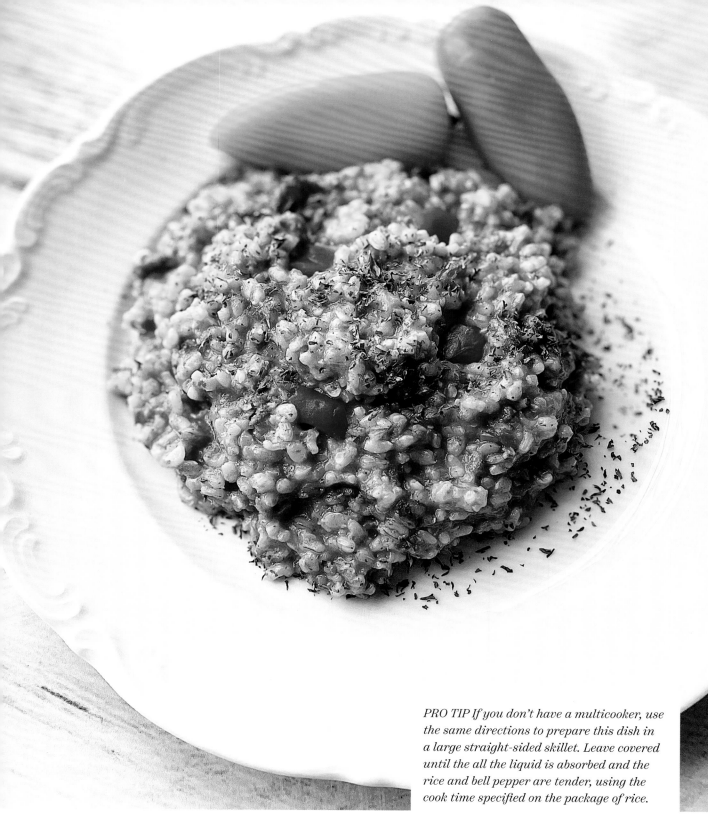

PRO TIP If you don't have a multicooker, use the same directions to prepare this dish in a large straight-sided skillet. Leave covered until the all the liquid is absorbed and the rice and bell pepper are tender, using the cook time specified on the package of rice.

CARIBBEAN JAMBALAYA

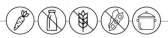

My one-pot version of this Creole entrée is a modern spin on a culinary recipe that has been popular since the 18th century. You know it's good eats when people are still clamoring for a dish after literally hundreds of years have gone by. One key difference here is the swapping of Cajun spices for a traditional Caribbean jerk seasoning. I recommend adding it in small increments, then continuing to add based on how much heat you can handle. (Jerk seasoning tends to be spice-forward when it first hits the tongue. It can be intense but is so delish!)

Ingredients

2 tablespoons (30 ml) olive oil, divided

1 cup (250 g) crumbled or chopped sausage (optional)

2 tablespoons (28 g) minced garlic

1½ cups (270 g) short grain brown or white rice, rinsed

1 cup (250 g) chopped red bell pepper

1 can (14.5 ounces [411 g]) diced tomatoes

2 cups (470 ml) water

1 cup (235 ml) vegetable broth

2 tablespoons (8 g) jerk seasoning

1½ (12 g) teaspoons salt

1 cup (240 ml) well-stirred coconut milk

¼ cup (61 g) pureed squash or pumpkin

6 ounces (170 g) medium precooked shrimp, thawed if frozen (optional)

1 tablespoon (30 ml) hot sauce (optional)

2 to 3 teaspoons (2 to 3 g) dried parsley, for garnish

Directions

1. Coat the bottom of a multicooker with 1 tablespoon (15 ml) oil.

2. Add the sausage, if using, and the garlic.

3. Add the rice, bell pepper, tomatoes with their juice, water, vegetable broth, jerk seasoning, salt, and the remaining oil.

4. Lock the lid in place, making sure the vent is sealed. Press the Pressure Cook (or Manual) button and set the timer for 23 minutes.

5. Once the time is up and your multicooker beeps, do a 5-minute natural release: let the timer reach 5 minutes, then press Cancel and carefully vent to release the steam.

6. Remove the lid and stir in the coconut milk and squash. Stir in the cooked shrimp, if using.

7. Adjust the seasoning if needed by adding more salt or hot sauce, if desired. Add some parsley on top before serving.

YIELD 6 Servings

PER SERVING 457 calories; 25 g fat; 11 g protein; 45 g carbohydrate

PREP TIME 10 mins **TOTAL TIME** 40 mins

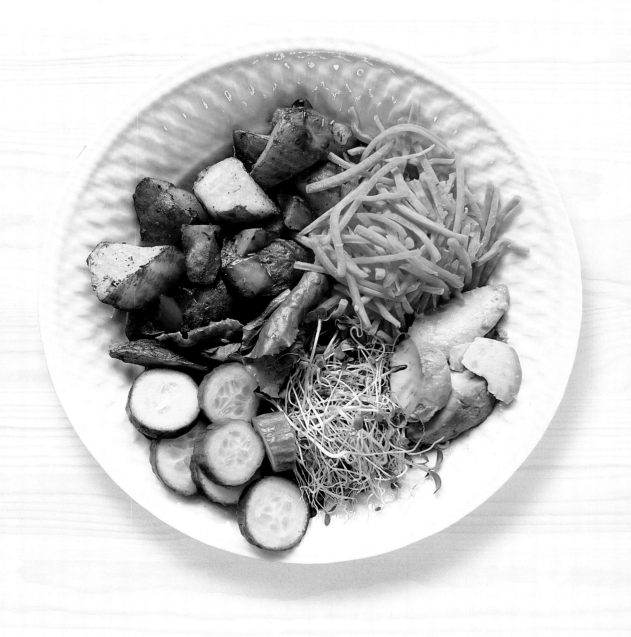

PRO TIP Bowls are excellent for meal prepping. You can pre-chop veggies and/or cook your protein in advance, so you can easily mix and match to create a new bowl each day. You can also meal prep completely assembled bowls if you prefer, but I like the ingredients approach for greater versatility.

THE ULTIMATE DIY BOWL

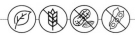

This one is more of a "template" than a recipe. However, once you get the basics down, you'll be able to easily recreate this *balanced* bowl with different ingredients again and again. It's also good to get into the habit of regularly combining raw and cooked foods, as nearly all foods lose a percentage of nutrient content if heated for enough time. I'm not suggesting you start eating uncooked potatoes, but pairing cooked potatoes with radishes, carrots, and other fresh produce will keep you steadily progressing toward meeting your carb ratio.

Ingredients

4 cups (about a 5- to 6-ounce [142 to 170 g] package) fresh greens (romaine, spinach, arugula, kale, sprouts, or a mix)

2 to 4 nutrient-dense veggies (carrots, cucumber, cabbage, beets, mushrooms, bell peppers, asparagus, radish, snap peas, green beans), raw, roasted, or grilled then chopped

Carbs (1 cup [250 g] cooked and diced red potatoes, sweet potatoes, or squash)

Proteins (1 cup [260 g] cooked beans, baked tofu, shredded roast chicken, or smoked salmon)

Healthy fats (½ cup [125 g] nuts, ¼ cup [56 g] pepitas, or 1 large avocado, sliced)

OPTIONAL TOPPINGS

Balsamic vinaigrette

Pesto

Tahini

Hummus

Salsa

Lime or lemon wedges

Directions

1. Divide the greens between two salad bowls.

2. Divide the remaining ingredients (veggies, carb, protein, and healthy fat) and top the leafy greens.

3. For an additional delicious flourish, drizzle with balsamic vinaigrette, pesto, tahini, hummus, or salsa and a spritz of lime or lemon.

YIELD 2 servings

PER SERVING varies depending on the ingredients

PREP TIME about 10 mins **TOTAL TIME** about 20 mins

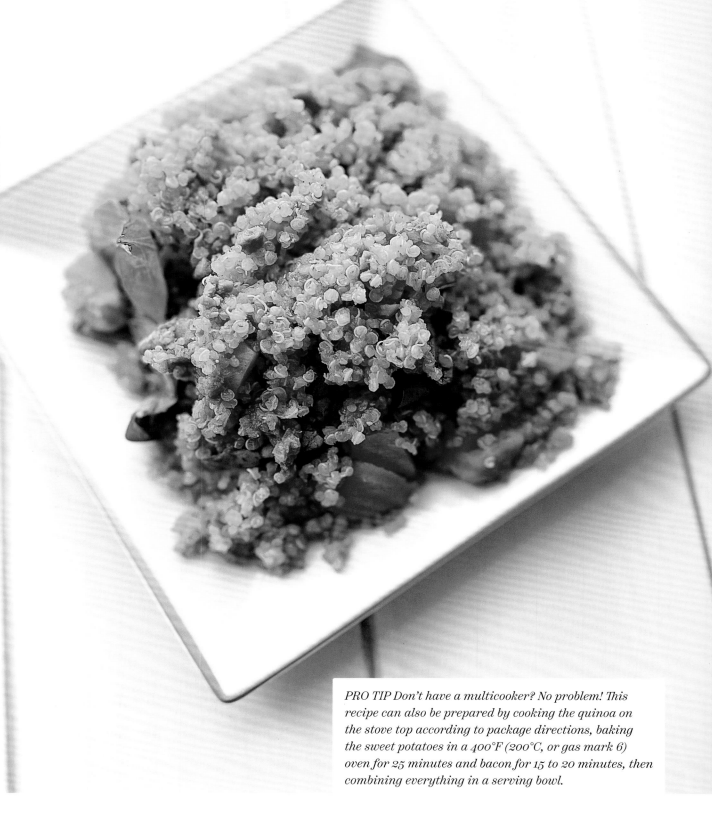

PRO TIP Don't have a multicooker? No problem! This recipe can also be prepared by cooking the quinoa on the stove top according to package directions, baking the sweet potatoes in a 400°F (200°C, or gas mark 6) oven for 25 minutes and bacon for 15 to 20 minutes, then combining everything in a serving bowl.

CAJUN "HOT HASH"

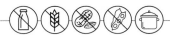

It is the best feeling when you finally get the flavor, texture, and visual aesthetic of a dish "just right." This is an entree I feel is well-suited for any time of day, and it can easily be doubled or tripled when you have a houseful of folks with different dietary preferences. The quinoa, sweet potato, and spinach make a scrumptious addition to scrambled eggs, shredded chicken, or plant-based crumbles.

Ingredients

Olive oil spray or nonstick cooking spray

3 cups (700 ml) water

2 cups (360 g) quinoa

1½ cups (375 g) frozen sweet potato cubes

8 strips bacon, diced or sliced

1 tablespoon (15 ml) maple syrup or (12 g) brown sugar

1 tablespoon (14 g) minced garlic

1 tablespoon (4 g) Cajun or taco seasoning

1 tablespoon (4 g) crushed red pepper flakes

3 cups (74 g) fresh spinach

2 tablespoons (30 ml) fresh lime juice (optional)

¼ cup (3 g) chopped fresh cilantro (optional)

Directions

1. Spray the bottom of a multicooker with olive oil spray.

2. Add the water and quinoa and stir.

3. Add the sweet potato, bacon, maple syrup, garlic, seasoning, and red pepper flakes.

4. Lock the lid in place, making sure the vent is sealed. Press the Pressure Cook (or Manual) button and set the timer for 5 minutes (it will take 6 to 8 minutes for the multicooker to pressurize before cooking begins).

5. Once the time is up and your multicooker beeps, allow to naturally release for 5 minutes (during the final "timing" phase), then release any remaining pressure. Carefully remove the lid once all the steam has escaped.

6. Stir in the spinach and lime juice, if using. Set the lid back on for 3 to 5 minutes, being careful to not let the greens completely wilt before serving.

7. Sprinkle with cilantro, if desired, once plated, along with more red pepper flakes or salt to taste.

YIELD 4 servings

PER SERVING 527 calories; 9 g fat; 37 g protein; 76 g carbohydrate

PREP TIME 5 mins **TOTAL TIME** 20 mins

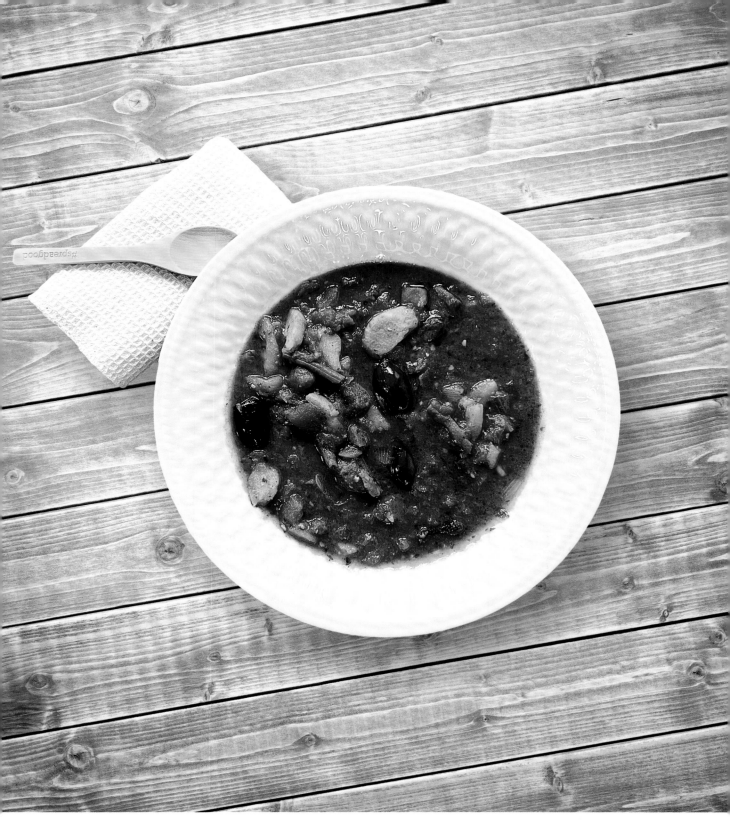

ESTOFADO ESPAÑOL

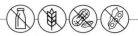

Having lived in five different countries, I have been lucky enough to meet numerous people enmeshed in the culinary and hospitality industries. Hence, this Spanish stew is so simple yet quite hearty—the exact meaning of the word *estofado*—and one of those dishes that is a perfect example of how you don't need to stand in front of the stove for hours, nor be wealthy, to eat *really* well daily.

Ingredients

1 tablespoon (15 ml) olive oil

1 pound (455 g) beef stew meat

2 teaspoons (3 g) sea salt

2 teaspoons (3 g) black pepper

1 can (14.5 ounces [411 g]) diced tomatoes

1 jar (12 ounces [340 g]) sofrito (see Pro Tip)

2 cups (454 g) chopped red potatoes

½ cup (125 g) chopped yellow onion

½ cup (125 g) pitted and halved black olives

4 ounces (113 g) fresh green beans (optional)

2 cloves garlic, minced

Directions

1. Heat the oil in a large skillet over medium heat.

2. Add the beef and sauté until it begins to brown on all sides. Season with the salt and pepper.

3. Transfer the beef and any pan juices to a slow cooker.

4. Add the tomatoes with their juice, sofrito, potatoes, onion, olives, green beans (if using), and garlic.

5. Cook on LOW until the beef and potatoes are fork-tender, 4 to 5 hours.

> *PRO TIP Sofrito is a popular seasoning used in Spain, Latin America, and the Caribbean. It can be purchased in dried form, as well as a liquid sauce.*

YIELD 6 servings

PER SERVING 343 calories; 20 g fat; 26 g protein; 17 g carbohydrate

PREP TIME 15 mins **TOTAL TIME** 4 to 5 hours

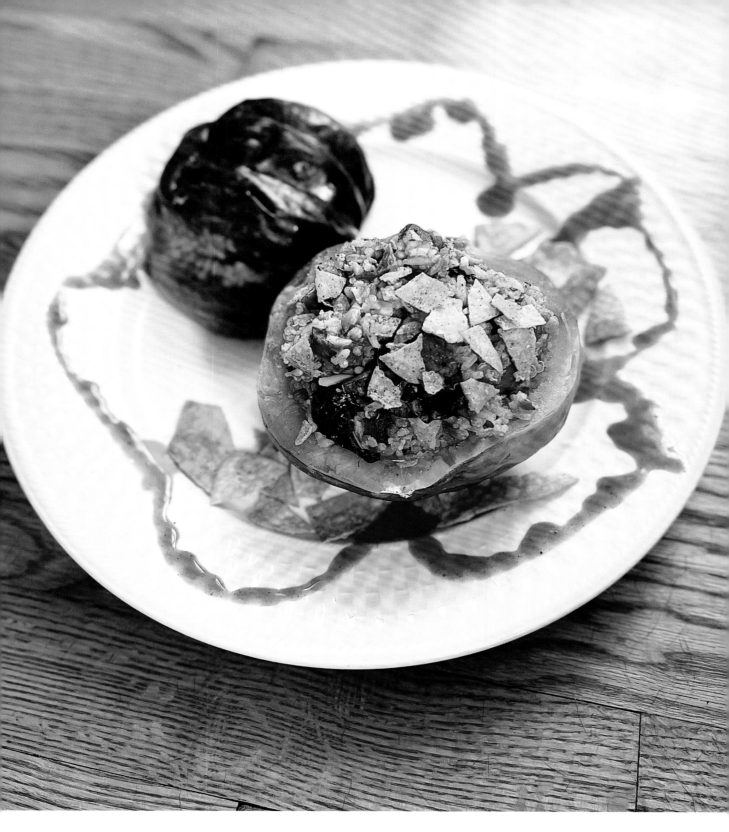

TEX-MEX STUFFED SQUASH

If you are worried about holiday or celebratory occasions being tricky to navigate while trying to stay within your target macro range, this "make and take" option won't look out of place (that is, it won't look *like diet food*) next to Aunt Sally's deviled eggs. Plus, the presentation alone is likely to tempt more than a few family members to join you for a taste test.

Ingredients

1 acorn squash, halved and seeded

1 cup (185 g) cooked quinoa or Mixed Grain Salad base (page 105)

1 cup (20 g) chopped kale

½ cup (112 g) prepared salsa

2 tablespoons (30 ml) olive oil

2 teaspoons (14 g) honey or (20 ml) maple syrup

¾ cup (187 g) frozen sweet corn (optional)

¼ cup (62 g) sliced smoked sausage or ½ cup (125 g) vegan chorizo (optional)

½ (120 ml) cup water

¼ cup (62 g) crushed tortilla chips, for garnish

Directions

1. Preheat the oven to 350°F (180°C, or gas mark 4).

2. Lightly oil the outside of each squash half and put in a baking dish.

3. In a bowl, mix the quinoa, kale, salsa, oil, and honey. Add in the corn and sausage or chorizo, if using.

4. Divide the mixture between the squash halves.

5. Add the water to the bottom of the baking dish before covering with aluminum foil. Bake until the squash is tender, about 45 minutes.

6. Serve immediately, topped with tortilla chips, if desired.

> *PRO TIP If you're meal prepping for the week, the Mixed Grain Salad recipe is great to use for the filling (double-check the grains used are gluten-free, if that's a concern). See the Meal Prep Planner (page 50) for more suggestions on meal prepping. Brown or white rice can also be subbed in for the quinoa to make this recipe gluten-free.*

YIELD 2 servings

PER SERVING 596 calories; 23 g fat; 19 g protein; 85 g carbohydrate

PREP TIME 15 mins **TOTAL TIME** 1 hour

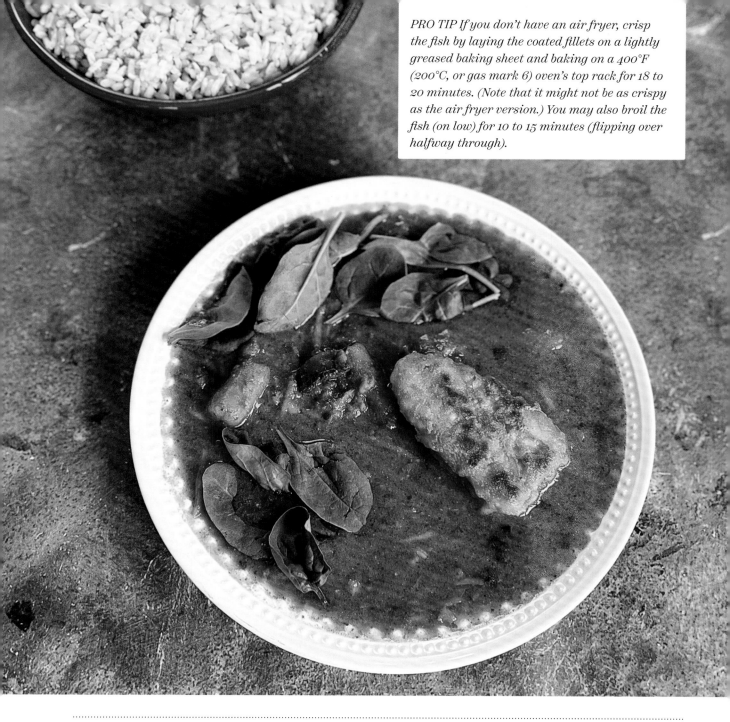

PRO TIP If you don't have an air fryer, crisp the fish by laying the coated fillets on a lightly greased baking sheet and baking on a 400°F (200°C, or gas mark 6) oven's top rack for 18 to 20 minutes. (Note that it might not be as crispy as the air fryer version.) You may also broil the fish (on low) for 10 to 15 minutes (flipping over halfway through).

YIELD 4 servings

PER SERVING 578 calories; 37 g fat; 15 g protein; 49 g carbohydrate

PREP TIME 5 mins **TOTAL TIME** 50 mins

CRISPY FISH CURRY

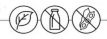

This recipe is wildly flexible! The base sauce goes with just about any morsel you choose to simmer in it. Thus, if you don't really dig onions, leave 'em out; toss in extra veggies; or use sweet potatoes instead of gold or red if that's all you have on hand. In fact, you can also omit the fish altogether to make this meal vegan.

Ingredients

FOR THE CURRY

2 tablespoons (30 ml) sesame oil

2 tablespoons (8 g) Indian curry powder or paste

1 tablespoon (8 g) ground cumin

1 cup (122 g) diced yellow onion

1 tablespoon (14 g) minced garlic

1 tablespoon (14 g) minced fresh ginger

6 small gold or red potatoes, cubed

2 large carrots, sliced or shredded

1 quart (1.1 L) vegetable broth, divided

1 can (13.5 ounces [400 ml]) coconut milk, well stirred

2 cups (56 g) fresh spinach, plus more for garnish

¼ cup (60 ml) fresh lime juice

1 teaspoon black pepper

Salt, to taste

4 cups (800 g) cooked brown rice, for serving (optional)

½ cup (6 g) fresh cilantro, chopped, for garnish

FOR THE FISH

4 whitefish fillets (4- to 6-ounces each), such as cod or tilapia, fresh or thawed

1 tablespoon (15 ml) olive oil

1 cup (112 g) bread crumbs

Directions

FOR THE CURRY

1. Warm the oil in a large pot over medium heat.

2. Add the curry powder and cumin and cook for about 30 seconds, stirring halfway through.

3. Add the onion, garlic, and ginger, and sauté until the onions start turning translucent, 4 to 5 minutes.

4. Add the potatoes and carrots. Stir well, cooking for 1 to 2 minutes.

5. Add half the veggie broth and cook for 20 minutes, partially covered.

6. Reduce the heat to low and stir in the coconut milk, along with the remaining veggie broth. Continue cooking until the potatoes and carrots are tender, 15 to 20 minutes more.

7. Add the spinach, lime juice, black pepper, and salt to taste.

8. Serve with cooked rice, if using, and set a piece of cooked fish on top. Garnish with a few spinach leaves or cilantro, if desired.

FOR THE FISH

1. After you add the coconut milk to the curry, start the fish by preheating an air fryer.

2. Coat the fish with the oil.

3. Put the bread crumbs on a small plate or in a bowl. Dredge each fillet in the bread crumbs, being sure to coat all sides.

4. Place the coated fish in the air fryer basket.

5. Cook at 390°F (200°C) for about 15 minutes, flipping over the fish halfway through cook time.

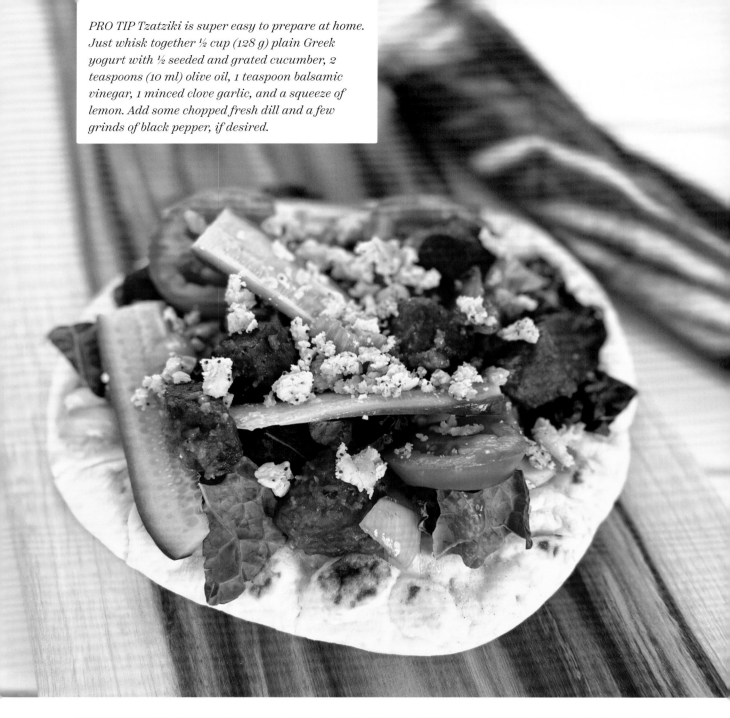

PRO TIP Tzatziki is super easy to prepare at home. Just whisk together ½ cup (128 g) plain Greek yogurt with ½ seeded and grated cucumber, 2 teaspoons (10 ml) olive oil, 1 teaspoon balsamic vinegar, 1 minced clove garlic, and a squeeze of lemon. Add some chopped fresh dill and a few grinds of black pepper, if desired.

YIELD 6 servings

PER SERVING 519 calories; 22g fat; 53 g protein; 28 g carbohydrate

PREP TIME 20 mins **TOTAL TIME** 6.5 hours or 1 hour 5 mins

ONE-POT GYROS

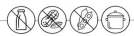

While working in Greece, gyros were one of the cheapest street foods I could afford on my "under the table" salary I earned running a hotel's pool bar. Working 10 to 12 hour days meant there were times I only ate one proper meal a day, and a gyro loaded with all the fixin's kept me fueled. It will similarly keep you going for whatever *endurance event* you've got on tap—whether it's three hours of running, court deliberations, or sports tournaments with the kids.

Ingredients

3 pounds (1.4 kg) beef chuck roast, large pieces of fat removed, meat sliced into thin ¼-inch strips

1 small red onion, chopped

3 tablespoons (45 ml) olive oil

2 teaspoons (5 g) garlic powder

1 teaspoon ground sage

1 teaspoon dried thyme

¾ teaspoon salt

6 soft pitas

2 cups (40 g) chopped kale

3 or 4 small plum tomatoes, sliced

1 or 2 small seedless cucumbers, sliced lengthwise

⅓ cup (37 g) regular or herbed crumbled feta cheese (optional)

¼ cup (60 ml) fresh lemon juice (optional)

Prepared tzatziki sauce (optional, see Pro Tip)

½ teaspoon freshly ground black pepper

Directions

IN A SLOW COOKER

1. Place the beef in a slow cooker with the chopped onions.

2. In a small bowl, combine the olive oil and spices, then add to the slow cooker.

3. Cover and cook on LOW for 6 hours, or until the beef is tender.

4. To serve, place the beef and kale leaves on each pita before topping with tomatoes and cucumber, plus feta, lemon juice, and a drizzle of tzatziki sauce, if using. Sprinkle with black pepper.

IN A MULTICOOKER

1. Follow steps 1 and 2, at left, placing the ingredients in a multicooker.

2. Secure the lid and confirm the valve is sealed. Press Manual or High Pressure, setting the timer for 30 minutes.

3. When time is up, let the pot sit for an additional 15 minutes before doing a manual pressure release. Carefully remove the lid.

4. Follow serving suggestions for step 4, at left.

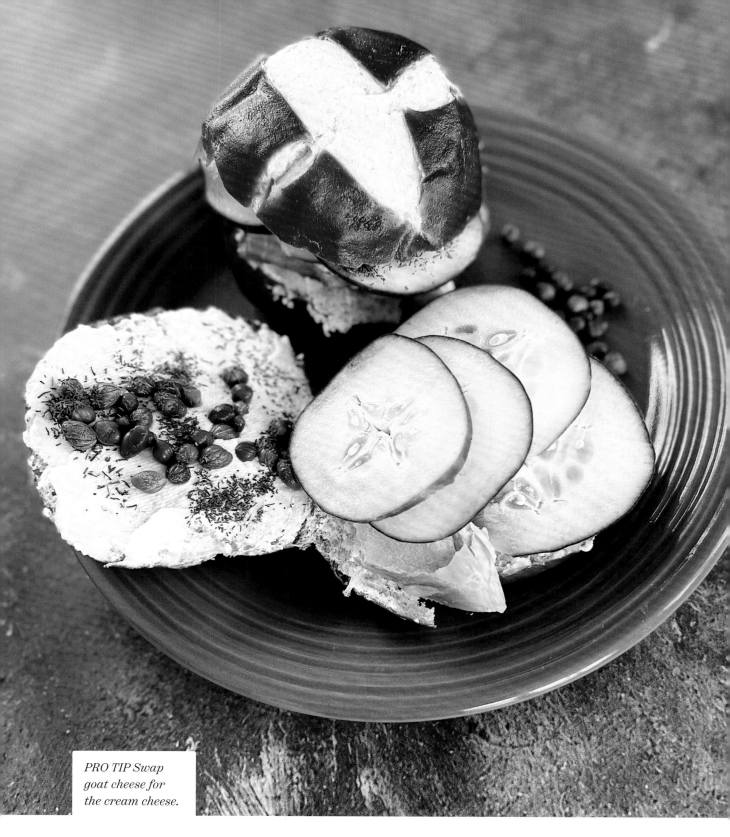

PRO TIP Swap goat cheese for the cream cheese.

SMOKED SALMON SLIDERS

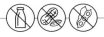

What's not to love about a properly nutritious nosh that requires zero cooking time or delivery fees? As long as you have all the ingredients on hand, you will have lunch or dinner on the table in less than 10 minutes. And swapping the buns for mini bagels transforms this into a luxe version of bagels & lox you can "wow" friends with over brunch.

Ingredients

6 mini pretzel or sandwich buns, halved

¼ cup (60 g) cream cheese (or dairy-free cream cheese)

1 package (3 ounces [85 g]) smoked salmon

1 medium cucumber, thinly sliced

3 teaspoons (12 g) dried dill

3 teaspoons (15 g) capers (optional)

Directions

1. Toast the bun halves.

2. For each slider, spread cream cheese on the top half of the bun.

3. Divide a third of the salmon between the bottom halves of two buns. Place 3 or 4 cucumber slices on each. Repeat with the remaining 4 buns, cucumbers, and salmon.

4. For every 2 sandwiches, sprinkle 1 teaspoon of the dill and 1 teaspoon capers, if using, on top of the cream cheese.

5. Put the two halves of the sandwich together then serve.

YIELD 3 servings

PER SERVING 280 calories; 11 g fat; 13 g protein; 33 g carbohydrate

PREP TIME 15 mins **TOTAL TIME** 15 mins

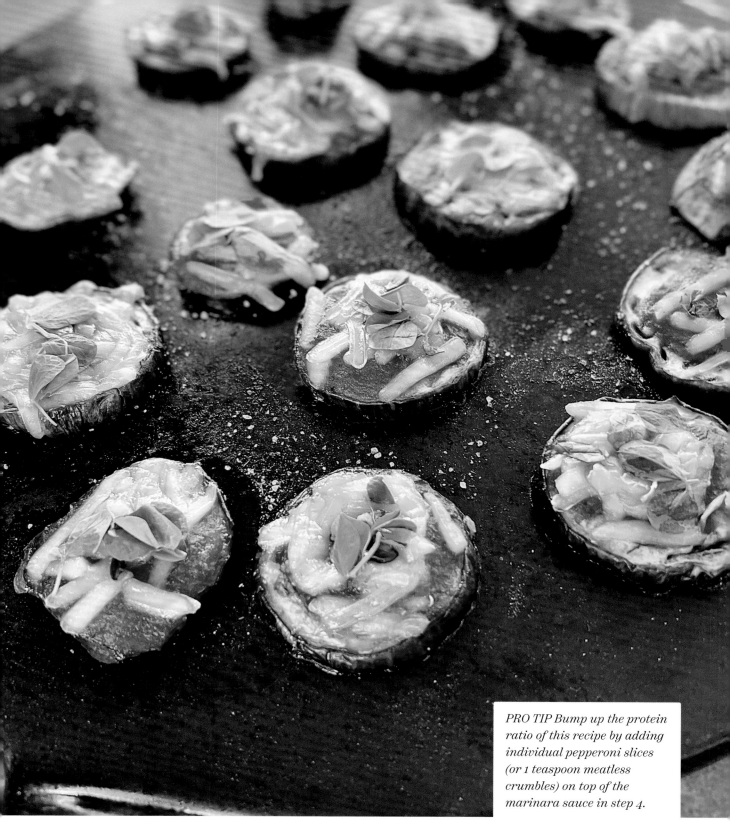

PRO TIP Bump up the protein ratio of this recipe by adding individual pepperoni slices (or 1 teaspoon meatless crumbles) on top of the marinara sauce in step 4.

CHEESY EGGPLANT ROUNDS

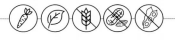

Pizza is a fave food of many, especially the "minis"... as in kiddos. The first time my daughter saw me assembling these in the kitchen, she requested I save her a few before heading off on a playdate. (And an eggplant fangirl *never* has she *ever* been). Making this your default recipe for when you're short on time, but still need a crowd-pleasing meal for all ages, is a wise choice.

Ingredients

4 tablespoons (60 ml) olive oil, divided

1 medium eggplant, thinly sliced ¼ cm to ½ cm thick

1 tablespoon (8 g) sea salt

1 tablespoon (8 g) black pepper

1 cup (250 g) prepared marinara sauce

1 cup (112 g) shredded Colby Jack cheese or dairy-free cheese

¼ cup (3 g) fresh basil leaves, for garnish

Directions

1. Preheat the oven to 400°F (200°C, or gas mark 6). Lightly coat a baking sheet or baking stone with half the oil.

2. Place the eggplant slices on the sheet in a single layer. Drizzle with the remaining oil and sprinkle with salt and pepper.

3. Bake until the eggplant is fully cooked, but the edges are slightly firm, about 20 minutes.

4. Spread about 1 tablespoon (15 g) marinara sauce on each eggplant slice and top with 3 to 4 teaspoons (17 g) of the cheese.

5. Set the oven to low broil and broil the eggplant until the cheese is melted, 3 to 5 minutes.

6. Garnish each round with a few leaves of fresh basil, if desired, before serving.

YIELD 6 to 8 servings (2 eggplant rounds each)

PER SERVING 148 calories; 11 g fat; 4 g protein; 9 g carbohydrate

PREP TIME 10 mins **TOTAL TIME** 40 mins

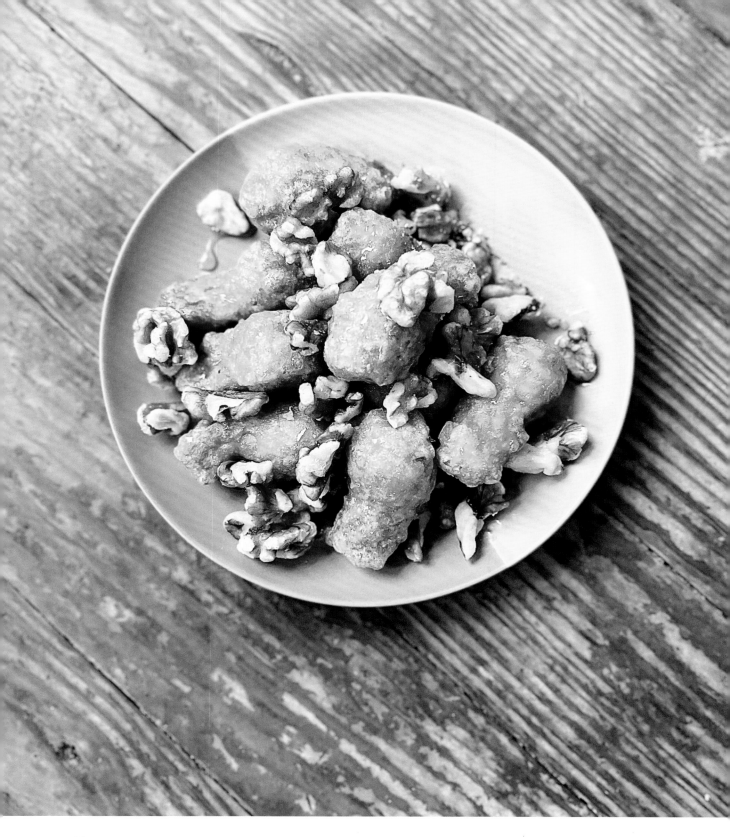

HONEY WALNUT CHICKEN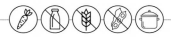

Adding sugar, salt, and crispiness to chicken is a foolproof dinner save every time. Try this homemade alternative to ordering takeout the next time you need a satisfying meal ASAP. Serve with Sheet Pan Sprouts and Spuds (page 107) or raw veggies like baby carrots, as a side.

Ingredients

1 pound (455 g) mini chicken wings (wingettes)

2 tablespoons (30 ml) olive oil or tea seed oil

2 teaspoons (9 g) baking powder

1 teaspoon salt

½ teaspoon black pepper

½ cup (170 g) honey

1 cup (4 ounces [112 g]) chopped walnuts

Directions

1. Preheat an air fryer to 380°F (190°C). Lightly coat the air fryer basket with some oil.

2. Put the wings in a bowl. Add the oil, baking powder, salt, and pepper. Toss to fully coat all the wings.

3. Place the seasoned chicken in a single layer in the air fryer basket and air fry for 15 minutes, flipping the wings once halfway through.

4. For an extra crispy skin, raise the temperature to 400°F (200°C) and air fry for 2 more minutes.

5. Use a digital meat thermometer to ensure the internal temperature is at least 165°F (75°C) before transferring the wings to a large plate in a pile.

6. Pour the honey over the wings, then generously cover with walnut pieces.

> *PRO TIP Substitute cauliflower florets for the chicken to make this recipe vegetarian. Cut the time in the air fryer in half.*

YIELD 4 servings (4 or 5 wings each)

PER SERVING 596 calories; 41 g fat; 25 g protein; 40 g carbohydrate

PREP TIME 10 mins **TOTAL TIME** 25 mins

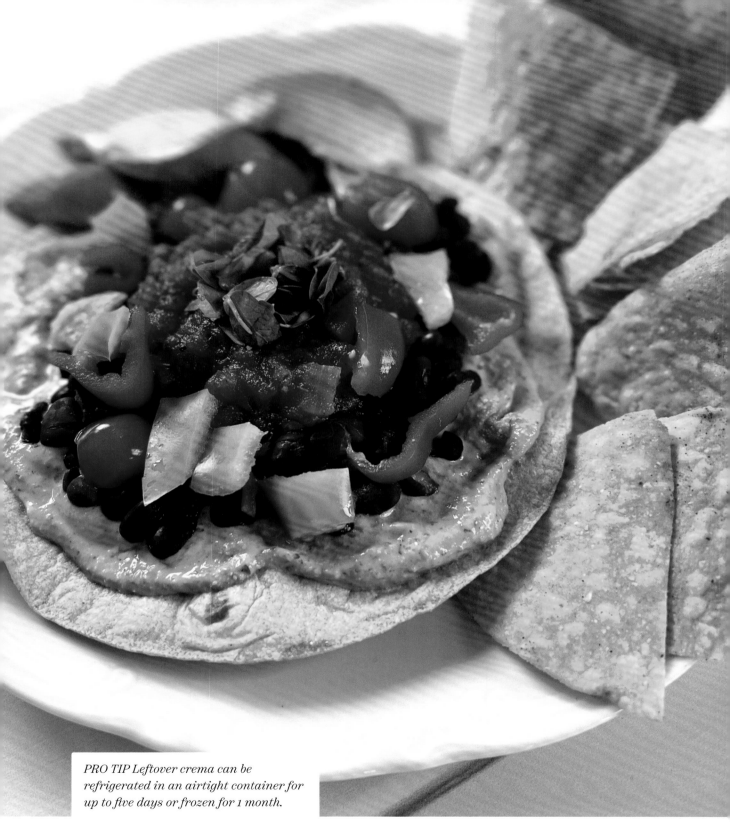

PRO TIP *Leftover crema can be refrigerated in an airtight container for up to five days or frozen for 1 month.*

BLACK BEAN TOSTADAS

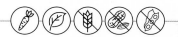

Tostada means "toast" in Spanish, so the "crisp" factor of the tortilla is essential to making sure this traditional Mexican dish turns out just right. But don't rush it! There's nothing worse than burning the base and having to start over.

Ingredients

TO MAKE THE CHIPOTLE CREMA (OPTIONAL)

1 cup (8 ounces [227 g]) vegan sour cream (or plain Greek yogurt)

2 tablespoons (40 g) ancho chile paste or chipotle-flavored hot sauce

2 tablespoons (30 ml) fresh lime juice

2 teaspoons (5 g) sea salt

TO MAKE THE TOSTADAS

4 flour or corn tortillas (6-inch [10-cm])

2 cups (365 g) cooked black beans or 1 can (15.5 ounces [439 g]), drained and rinsed

1½ tablespoons (21 g) minced garlic

1½ tablespoons (12 g) paprika

2 teaspoons (5 g) salt

8 tablespoons (120 ml) Chipotle Crema (see above) or 112 g shredded Cheddar cheese

1 cup (225 g) prepared salsa

1 medium tomato, chopped

1 small red bell pepper, chopped

1 small yellow bell pepper, chopped

1 medium lime

1 medium avocado, sliced (optional)

Tortilla chips (optional)

¼ cup (3 g) fresh basil or cilantro, for garnish

Directions

1. If using the Chipotle Crema, stir together all the ingredients in a small bowl until smooth. Chill for at least 30 minutes prior to using.

2. Preheat the oven to 350°F (180°C, or gas mark 4). Place 2 tortillas side-by-side in 2 oven-safe skillets, or set all 4 on a baking stone or baking sheet.

3. Bake until crisp, about 15 minutes, flipping over halfway through.

4. Meanwhile, in a small saucepan, combine the beans with the garlic, paprika, and salt. Gently heat over medium-low until warm. (Alternatively, heat in the microwave in a microwave-safe dish.)

5. To assemble, spread 2 tablespoons (30 ml) of the Chipotle Crema, or sprinkle 2 tablespoons (28 g) cheese, on each tortilla. Top with equal portions of the beans, salsa, tomato, and peppers.

6. Add a spritz of fresh lime juice as a final flourish, along with the avocado, tortilla chips, and basil or cilantro, if using.

YIELD 4 servings

PER SERVING 360 calories; 14 g fat; 12 g protein; 50 g carbohydrate

PREP TIME 15 mins **TOTAL TIME** 30 mins

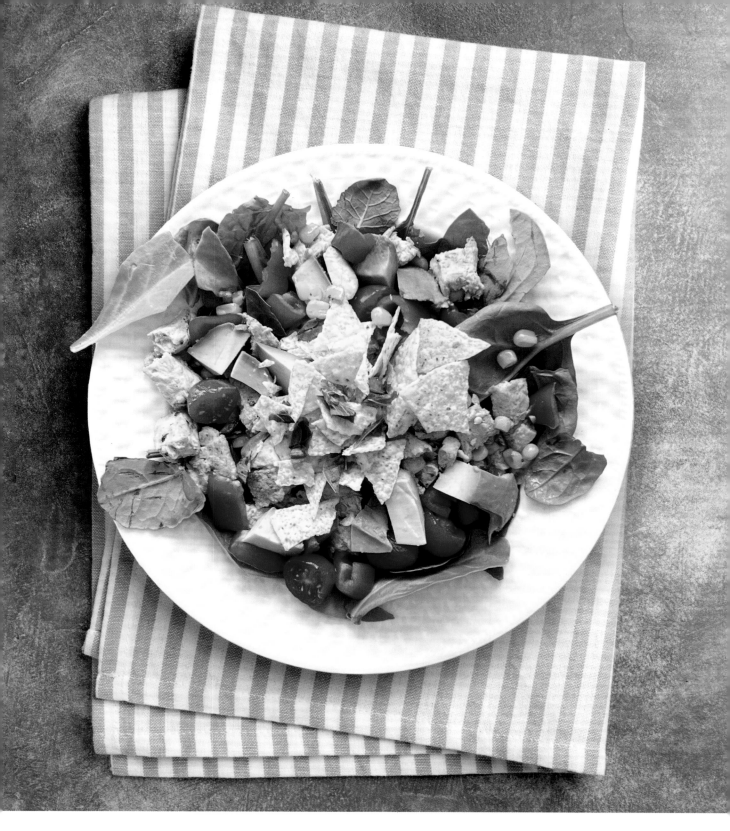

CILANTRO LIME CHICKEN SALAD

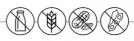

During the warmer months, when a large variety of veggies and leafy greens are in season, I eat salad for at least one meal most weekdays. Meals like this really make prepping ingredients at the start of the week well worth it because no matter how crunched for time I feel, I know there's nutritious, delish food ready and waiting in the fridge.

Ingredients

2 chicken breasts (4 ounces [115 g] each)

1 container (5 ounces [142 g]) mixed salad greens or prewashed lettuce

½ cup (61 g) diced bell peppers (red, yellow, orange)

¼ cup (30 g) diced red onion

½ cup (142 g) halved grape tomatoes

¼ cup (37 g) sweet corn

1 large avocado, sliced

¼ cup (62 g) crushed tortilla chips

2 tablespoons (30 ml) fresh lime juice

2 tablespoons (2 g) fresh cilantro

¼ cup (56 g) prepared salsa verde (optional)

Directions

1. Prepare the chicken by pan-frying or grilling until cooked through. Once cool enough to handle, cut into strips.

2. Divide the salad greens between two bowls.

3. Evenly divide all the veggies between the bowls, adding in a few strips of chicken while doing so.

4. Top each salad with half the tortilla chips, lime juice, and cilantro.

5. Add 2 tablespoons (23 g) salsa verde, if desired, to each bowl as the final flourish.

YIELD 2 servings

PER SERVING 439 calories; 27 g fat; 22 g protein; 33 g carbohydrate

PREP TIME 20 mins **TOTAL TIME** 30 mins

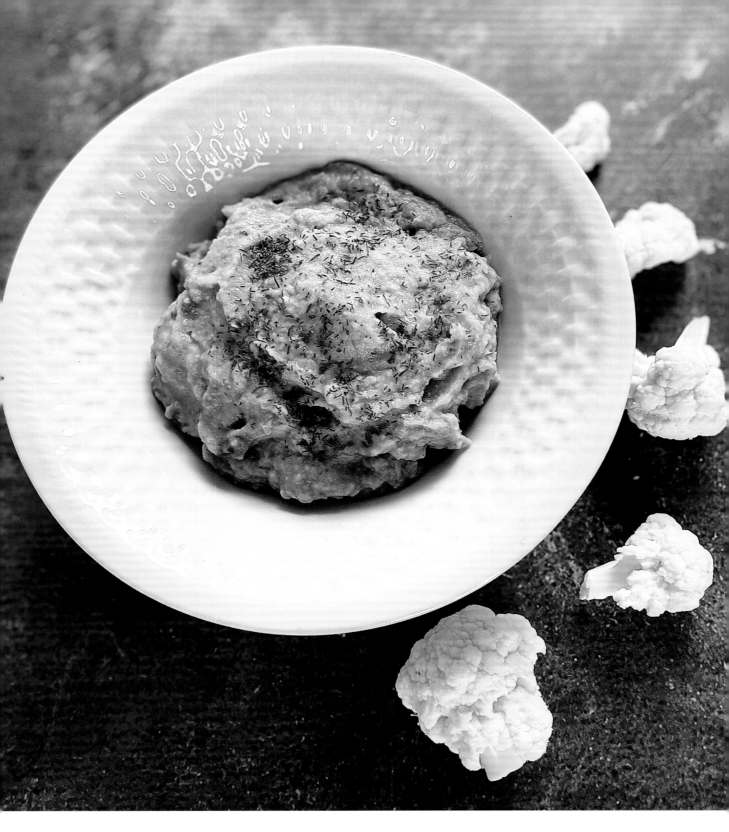

CAULIFLOWER MASHED "TATERS"

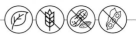

This is an excellent side to add into your potluck rotation because it's low maintenance in terms of cost, hands-on labor, and stress for gatherings where one or more people have food allergies. Also, if you suddenly have an intense craving for mashed potatoes, this is a low-carb alternative to that classic nosh.

Ingredients

2 heads cauliflower, cut into florets

2 tablespoons (30 ml) skim milk or dairy-free milk (optional)

2 tablespoons (30 ml) olive oil

2 tablespoons (8 g) dried dill

1 teaspoon salt

¾ teaspoon black pepper, or to taste

Directions

1. Steam or boil the cauliflower until fully tender, 10 to 15 minutes. Drain, if necessary, and transfer to a large bowl.

2. For a thicker mash, use a fork and a wooden spoon to mash the cauliflower with the milk (if using), oil, dill, salt, and pepper.

3. For a smoother texture, purée the cauliflower with the remaining ingredients in a food processor or blender for 30 seconds to 1 minute, until desired consistency is reached. Transfer to a serving bowl.

4. Sprinkle additional dill on top before serving, if desired.

> *PRO TIP This dish is great to make ahead! Reheat in a covered oven-safe dish at 350°F [180°C, or gas mark 4] for about 15 minutes.*

YIELD 6 servings

PER SERVING 121 calories; 5 g fat; 6 g protein; 16 g carbohydrate

PREP TIME 10 mins **TOTAL TIME** 30 mins

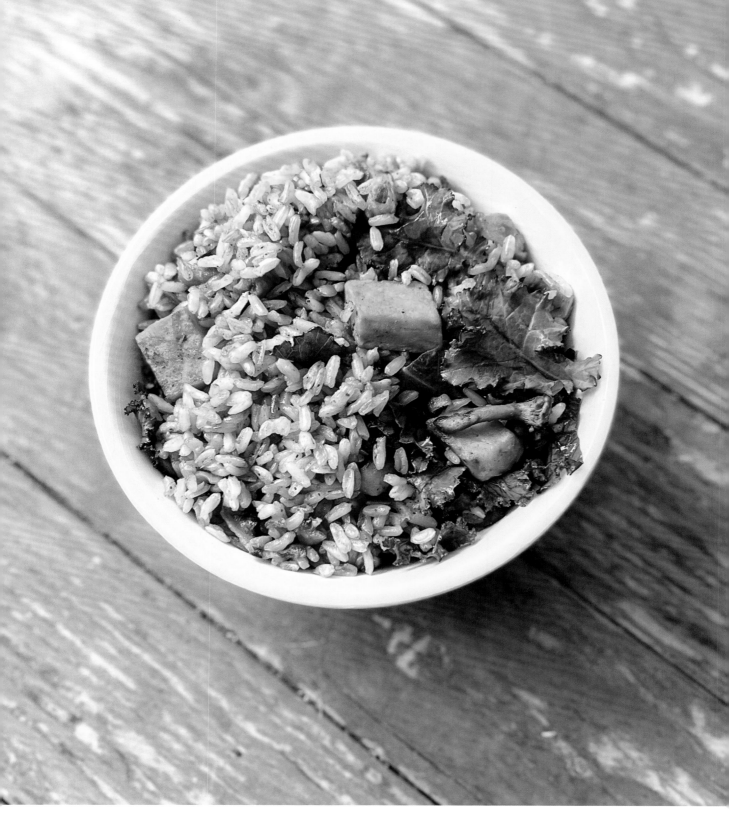

HARVEST RICE

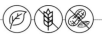

My baked rendition of fried rice leans into the veggies that are typically in season where I live come fall. It's also a flexible meal prep staple: as long as you have a few cups of rice on hand, plus two or three vegetables already chopped and waiting in the fridge, this meal can be thrown together while the oven preheats. You can even toss in leftover proteins like steak or seitan—whatever happens to be in your fridge.

Ingredients

2 cups (about 1 lb [454 g]) cubed sweet potatoes

3 tablespoons (45 ml) sesame oil, divided

2 tablespoons (30 ml) liquid aminos (or 1 tablespoon tamari or soy sauce)

3 cloves garlic, minced

1 tablespoon (8 g) black pepper

3 cups (540 g) brown or wild rice

1 cup (about 2 ounces [56 g]) oyster or shitake mushrooms, stemmed (optional)

3 cups (700 ml) vegetable or chicken broth

1½ cups (350 ml) water

3 cups (60 g) chopped kale

2 tablespoons (28 g) pepitas, for garnish

Directions

1. Preheat the oven to 350°F (180°C, or gas mark 4).

2. In a bowl, toss the sweet potatoes with 1 tablespoon of the oil, the liquid aminos, garlic, and pepper.

3. Rinse the rice thoroughly then transfer to an 8-inch (20-cm) square or 9 x 13-inch (23 x 33-cm) baking dish. Spread evenly.

4. Spread the sweet potatoes and mushrooms (if using) over the rice. Be sure the veggie(s) fully form a top layer.

5. Add the broth, water, and the remaining 2 tablespoons oil to the baking dish.

6. Bake until the rice is completely cooked and the sweet potatoes are browned and tender, 35 to 40 minutes. Remove from the oven, mix in the kale, and let sit for 5 minutes before dishing up.

7. Add 1 teaspoon pepitas on top of individual servings, if desired.

YIELD 6 servings

PER SERVING 486 calories; 10 g fat; 13 g protein; 87 g carbohydrate

PREP TIME 10 mins **TOTAL TIME** 50 mins

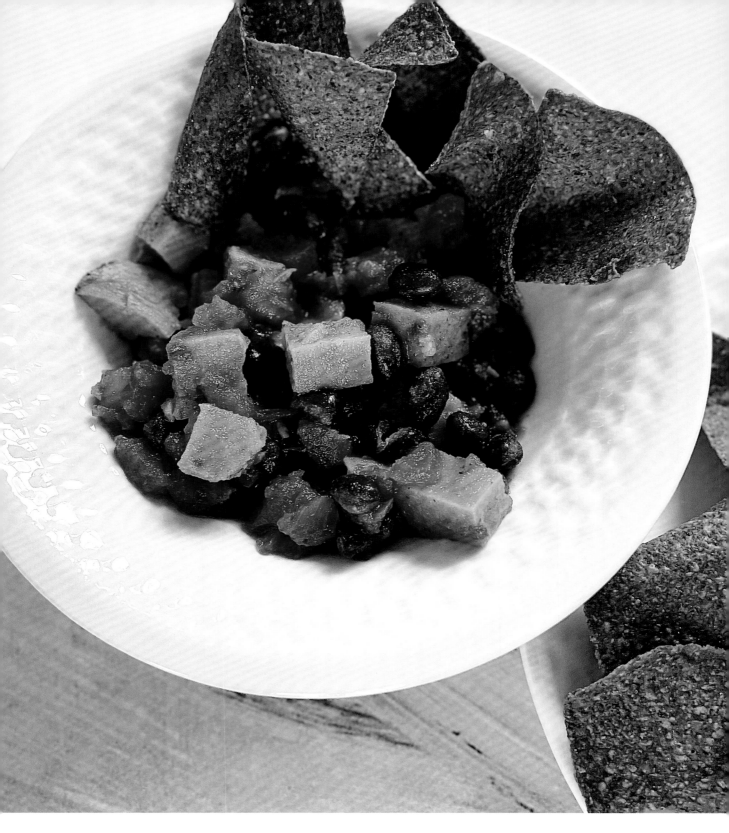

LOADED SWEET POTATO SALSA

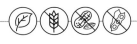

Toss in fresh leafy greens to upgrade this delectable dip into a salad. But go easy on the spice when mixing this up for a crowd; the cayenne can always be left on the side as a self-serve option.

Ingredients

4 large sweet potatoes, peeled (if desired) and cut into small cubes

1 cup (122 g) diced onion

2 tablespoons (30 ml) olive oil

1 tablespoon (8 g) garlic powder

2 teaspoons (5 g) paprika

Cayenne pepper, to taste (optional)

2 cups (365 g) cooked black beans or 1 can (15.5 ounces [439 g]), drained and rinsed

1 can (14.5 ounces [411 g]) diced tomatoes, drained

3 to 4 tablespoons (12 to 16 g) taco seasoning or chili powder

3 tablespoons (45 ml) fresh lime juice

Tortilla chips, for serving

Directions

1. Preheat the oven to 400°F (200°C, or gas mark 6).

2. Put the sweet potatoes on a baking sheet along with the onions, oil, garlic powder, paprika, and a dash of cayenne, if using. Toss to coat, then spread evenly in a single layer before baking for 20 minutes.

3. Meanwhile, in a large bowl, combine the beans, tomatoes, taco seasoning, and lime juice. Stir well.

4. After 20 minutes, take the potatoes out of the oven. Add the black beans to the sweet potatoes and carefully stir together before returning to the oven for an additional 10 minutes.

5. Serve with tortilla chips (or mixed greens, if opting for the salad version).

YIELD 10 servings

PER SERVING 146 calories; 0 g fat; 5 g protein; 31 g carbohydrate

PREP TIME 15 mins **TOTAL TIME** 50 mins

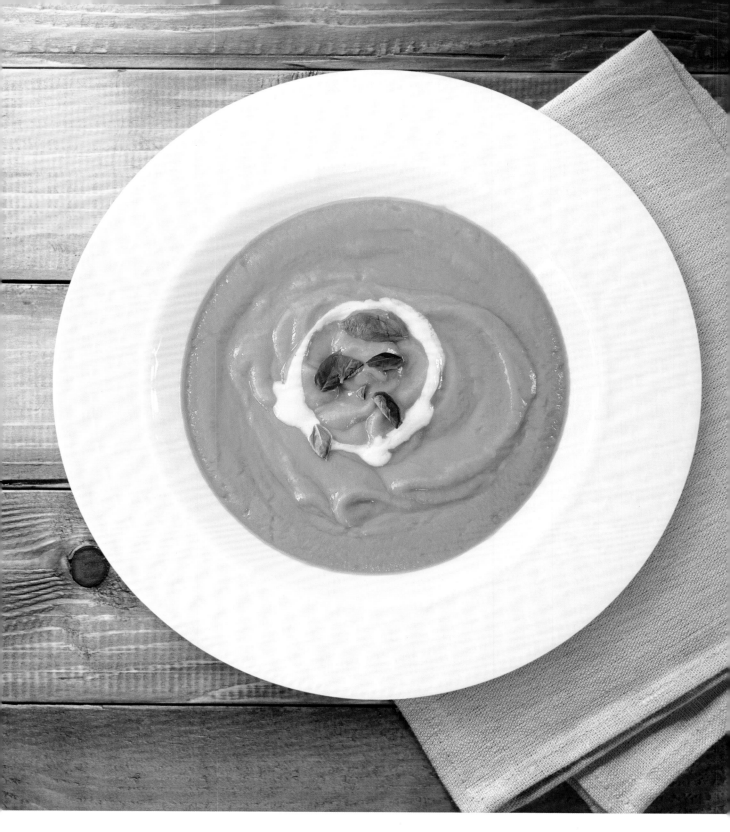

CARROT GINGER BISQUE

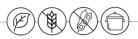

I am the kind of person who can eat soup any time of year, doesn't matter what the temperature is outdoors or which produce is currently in large supply at the local farmer's market. Thus, you can swap an alternate main vegetable as the base ingredient for a "no fuss" variation on the OG specs below. I've subbed in pureed pumpkin, squash, or sweet potatoes with great success, and the fact that it's made in the slow cooker means I can have this in the summer without breaking a sweat in the kitchen.

Ingredients

2 cups (470 ml) low-sodium vegetable broth

2 cups (470 ml) water

8 large carrots, sliced

1 cup (122 g) chopped yellow onion

1 cup (122 g) chopped celery

3 tablespoons (36 g) brown sugar

2 tablespoons (30 ml) olive oil

1 tablespoon (14 g) minced fresh ginger

1 tablespoon (8 g) ground cinnamon

2 teaspoons (5 g) ground cloves

1 teaspoon salt

1 cup (240 ml) well-stirred coconut milk

¼ cup (60 g) low-fat or nondairy yogurt (optional)

¼ cup (3 g) small basil leaves or chopped parsley, for garnish

Directions

1. To a slow cooker, add the broth, water, carrots, onion, celery, brown sugar, oil, ginger, cinnamon, cloves, and salt.

2. Cover and cook on HIGH for 90 minutes (or on LOW for 3 hours).

3. Let cool for 20 minutes, then add the coconut milk.

4. Purée the soup using an immersion blender. (Alternatively, carefully transfer the soup to a blender, in batches if necessary, and purée until smooth.)

5. Add a drizzle of yogurt and/or a sprinkle of basil or parsley before serving, if desired.

> PRO TIP Double the recipe then divide into 2 to 3-serving portions to freeze in airtight containers for up to 2 months. Defrost and use as needed.

YIELD 4 servings

PER SERVING 226 calories; 13 g fat; 3 g protein; 28 g carbohydrate

PREP TIME 15 mins **TOTAL TIME** 2.5 to 4 hours

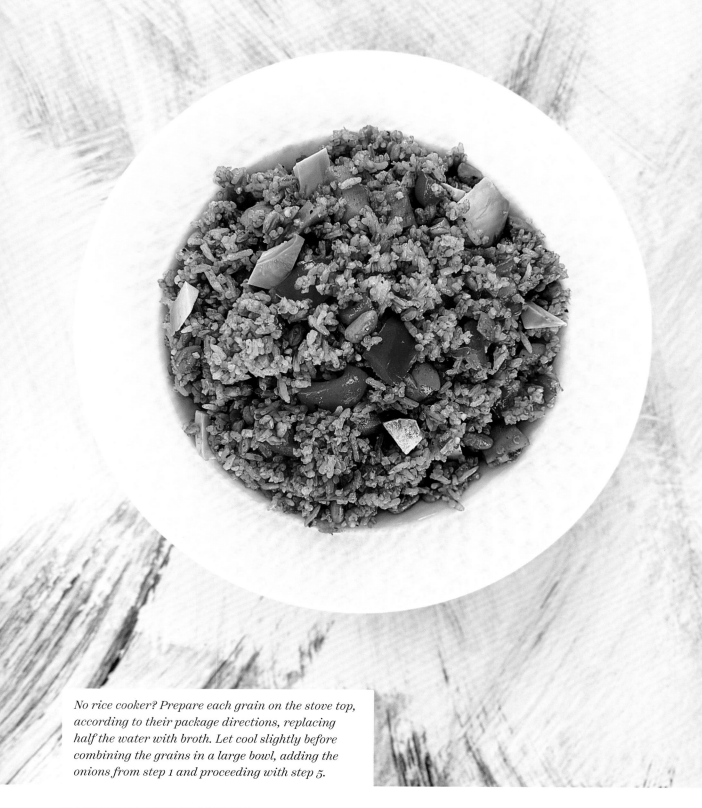

No rice cooker? Prepare each grain on the stove top, according to their package directions, replacing half the water with broth. Let cool slightly before combining the grains in a large bowl, adding the onions from step 1 and proceeding with step 5.

MIXED GRAIN SALAD

As an avid runner, I know how important it is to have enough "gas in the tank" come race day, but carb loading can be done sans chowing down on pasta. Which is why you should incorporate at least three different whole grains when making this salad if you're training for a strength-based competition and/or doing high-intensity cardio workouts more than four days a week. This recipe also makes great use of the rice cooker—it cooks all the grains at once.

Ingredients

2 tablespoons (30 ml) olive oil

½ cup (61 g) diced onion

1 cup (180 g) quinoa

1 cup (180 g) white or brown rice

1 cup (180 g) farro

2 cups (470 ml) vegetable or chicken broth

2 cups (470 ml) water

2 tablespoons (30 ml) maple syrup or molasses

2 tablespoons (16 g) ground turmeric

1 tablespoon (15 ml) tamari or soy sauce

1 tablespoon (15 g) Harissa or chili garlic sauce

1 tablespoon (14 g) minced garlic

2 teaspoons (3 g) dried basil or thyme

1 cup (122 g) chopped red bell pepper

¾ cup (188 g) pitted olives

1 large avocado, cubed

½ cup (70 g) cooked shredded chicken (optional)

Directions

1. Heat the oil in large saucepan over medium-high heat. Add the onions and sauté until translucent, 4 to 5 minutes. If you don't have a rice cooker, jump to the Pro Tip before proceeding to the next step.

2. Add the quinoa, rice, and farro to the onions, stirring to coat.

3. Transfer to a rice cooker and add the broth and water before turning on.

4. When the cook time is complete, unplug the rice cooker.

5. Stir in the maple syrup, turmeric, tamari, Harissa, garlic, and basil. Let cool slightly.

6. Mix in the bell pepper, olives, avocado, and chicken (if using) immediately before serving.

YIELD 6 servings

PER SERVING 424 calories; 22 g fat; 11 g protein; 51 g carbohydrate

PREP TIME 10 mins **TOTAL TIME** 1 hour

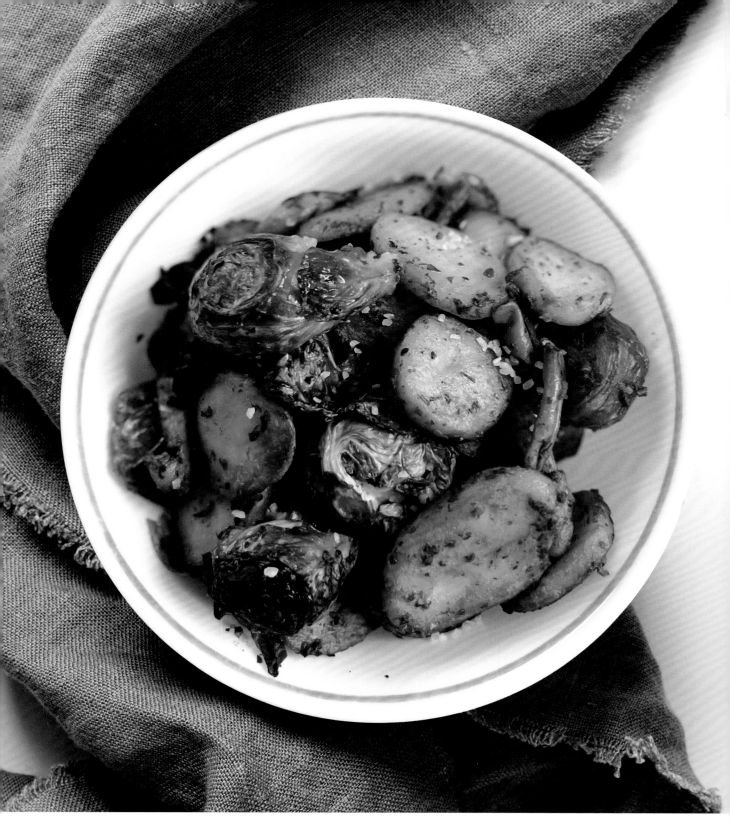

SHEET PAN SPROUTS AND SPUDS

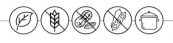

Another easy-peasy side! However, make sure the sprout and potato pieces are cut similar in size and thickness so they cook relatively at the same speed. Add sliced breakfast sausage to make this an ideal addition to a brunch spread.

Ingredients

4 tablespoons (60 ml) olive oil or tea seed oil, divided

2 pounds (910 g) small gold or red potatoes, cut into rounds

1 pound (455 g) Brussels sprouts, trimmed and halved

1 tablespoon (8 g) sea salt

3 cloves garlic, minced

1 tablespoon (8 g) black pepper

1 tablespoon (4 g) dried dill

2 teaspoons (5 g) onion powder

1 teaspoon ground sage

½ teaspoon dried parsley (optional)

Directions

1. Preheat the oven to 400°F (200°C, or gas mark 6). Use 1 tablespoon (15 ml) of the oil to grease a baking sheet.

2. Add the potatoes, Brussels sprouts, the remaining 3 tablespoons oil, and spices (except the parsley) to the baking sheet. Toss until the veggies are well coated then spread in an even layer.

3. Bake for 25 minutes, stir the veggies, then bake until the potatoes are fork tender, an additional 20 to 25 minutes.

4. Serve warm, sprinkled with parsley, if desired.

YIELD 6 servings

PER SERVING 220 calories; 9 g fat; 6 g protein; 31 g carbohydrate

PREP TIME 15 mins **TOTAL TIME** 1 hour

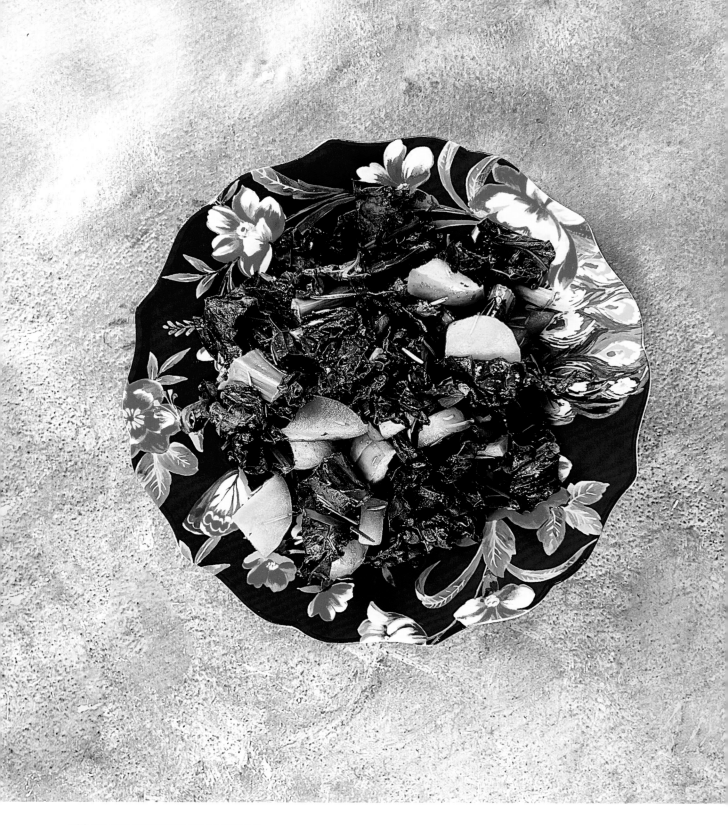

OVEN-BAKED APPLES AND KALE

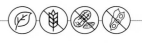

Here is a dairy-free and low-sodium side that bests green bean casserole in terms of nutrients. Cut. Combine. Season. Bake. It really is that easy. And don't shy away from the number of compliments you're likely to get for fare that required such a minimal amount of work. Whoever said "good" must be acquainted with "hard" in the kitchen? Certainly not me!

Ingredients

3 large apples, cored and chopped

¼ cup (30 g) chopped red onion

¼ cup (60 ml) balsamic vinegar

2 tablespoons (30 ml) olive oil

1 tablespoon (15 g) Dijon mustard

1 teaspoon salt

1 teaspoon black pepper

6 cups (120 g) torn fresh kale

Directions

1. Preheat the oven to 375°F (190°C, or gas mark 5).

2. In a large bowl, toss together the apples, onions, vinegar, oil, mustard, salt, and pepper.

3. Transfer the mixture to a baking sheet in a single layer and bake for 15 to 20 minutes.

4. Remove from the oven and add the kale, stirring it and the apples together before returning to the oven.

5. Bake until the kale is crisp along the edges, another 8 to 10 minutes. Let cool slightly before serving.

YIELD 4 servings (about 1 cup each)

PER SERVING 154 calories; 7 g fat; 2 g protein; 23 g carbohydrate

PREP TIME 10 mins **TOTAL TIME** 35 mins

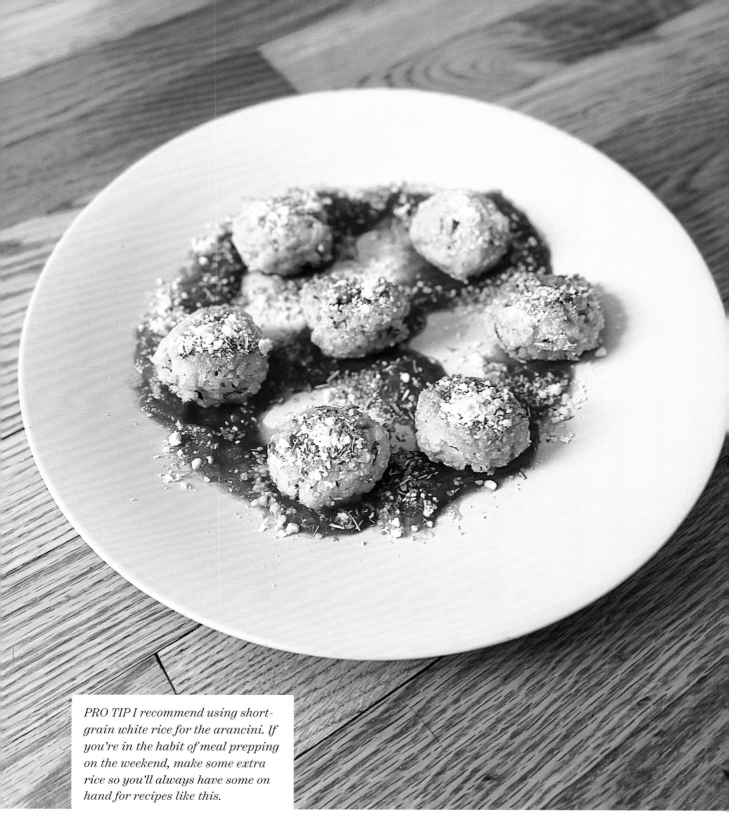

PRO TIP I recommend using short-grain white rice for the arancini. If you're in the habit of meal prepping on the weekend, make some extra rice so you'll always have some on hand for recipes like this.

ZUCCHINI ARANCINI

Hands down, this is the most time-consuming recipe in this book, but the payoff is HUGE. You won't regret a single moment you spent in the kitchen after your first bite into one of these crispy, tasty morsels. Arancini are Italian rice balls usually stuffed with other ingredients, such as cheese, then deep fried. My version has more of a Cali cuisine vibe courtesy of a fresh veggie, gluten-free batter, and a light pan sear.

Ingredients

1 cup (186 g) cooked rice (see Pro Tip)

½ cup (85 g) shredded zucchini

¾ cup (92 g) oat flour

2 eggs (or equivalent egg substitute)

2 cloves garlic, minced

2 teaspoons (5 g) salt

2 teaspoons (5 g) black pepper

1 cup (152 g) cornmeal

2 tablespoons (30 ml) olive oil

½ cup (125 g) prepared marinara sauce (optional)

⅓ cup (28 g) grated Parmesan cheese (optional)

Directions

1. In a medium bowl, combine the rice and zucchini.

2. Add the flour, 1 egg (or half the egg substitute), the garlic, salt, and pepper, mixing until evenly combined.

3. Roll into 12 small balls and set aside.

4. In a small bowl, whisk the remaining egg.

5. Lightly beat the remaining egg or egg substitute in a small bowl, and spread the cornmeal on a large plate.

6. Dip each rice ball into the egg, then roll in the cornmeal. Set aside until all are coated.

7. Heat 1 tablespoon (15 ml) of the oil in a large skillet over medium heat. Add half the coated rice balls and cook until golden on all sides, 8 to 10 minutes. Rotate at least twice for even cooking.

8. Remove from the skillet and repeat with the remaining balls and oil.

9. Serve warm with the marinara sauce and/or Parmesan cheese.

YIELD 4 servings

PER SERVING 435 calories; 6 g fat; 12 g protein; 83 g carbohydrate

PREP TIME 15 mins **TOTAL TIME** 35 mins

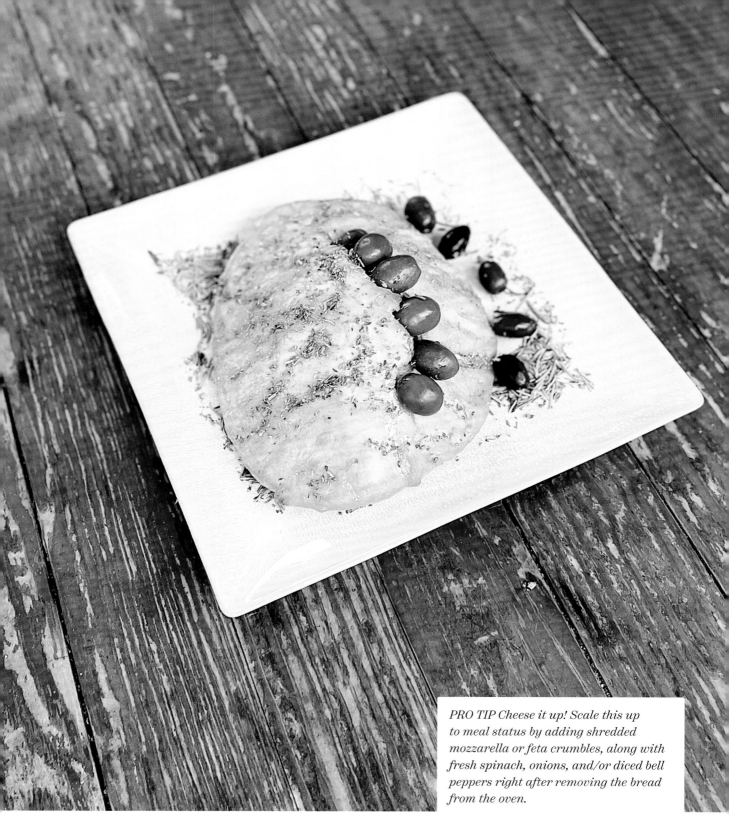

PRO TIP Cheese it up! Scale this up to meal status by adding shredded mozzarella or feta crumbles, along with fresh spinach, onions, and/or diced bell peppers right after removing the bread from the oven.

OLIVE FOCACCIA

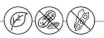

Homemade bread is one of life's simple luxuries. What makes this recipe even better is that it requires no yeast. Eliminating any "rising time" means it's totally feasible to bake—and eat— this all within your lunch hour, if you're working from home. Also, using a baking stone for this recipe helps ensure the bottom of the focaccia cooks evenly.

Ingredients

3 tablespoons (45 ml) olive oil, divided

2 cups (280 g) all-purpose flour, plus a little extra for dusting

1 tablespoon (14 g) baking powder

2 teaspoons (5 g) sea salt

1 teaspoon minced garlic

1 cup (235 ml) water

Coarse sea salt

¼ cup (62 g) pitted olives

2 to 3 tablespoons (8 to 12 g) crushed dried rosemary

Directions

1. Preheat the oven to 425°F (220°C, or gas mark 7).

2. Grease a baking stone or baking sheet with 1 tablespoon (15 ml) of the oil.

3. In a large bowl, combine the flour, baking powder, salt, and garlic before mixing in the water and 1 tablespoon of the oil.

4. Turn the dough out onto a lightly floured surface and knead until a ball of dough comes together, about 2 minutes.

5. Put the dough on the baking stone and shape into a ½-inch (1 cm)-thick rectangle or round. Using your fingertips, poke indentations into the top of the dough.

6. Spread the remaining 1 tablespoon olive oil over the dough and sprinkle coarse sea salt across the top.

7. Bake until it begins to turn golden brown, about 25 minutes.

8. Remove from oven and let cool slightly before placing the olives into the indentations. Dust the rosemary over the top.

9. Cut into 6 pieces before serving.

YIELD 6 servings

PER SERVING 232 calories; 9 g fat; 4 g protein; 32 g carbohydrate

PREP TIME 10 mins **TOTAL TIME** 35 mins

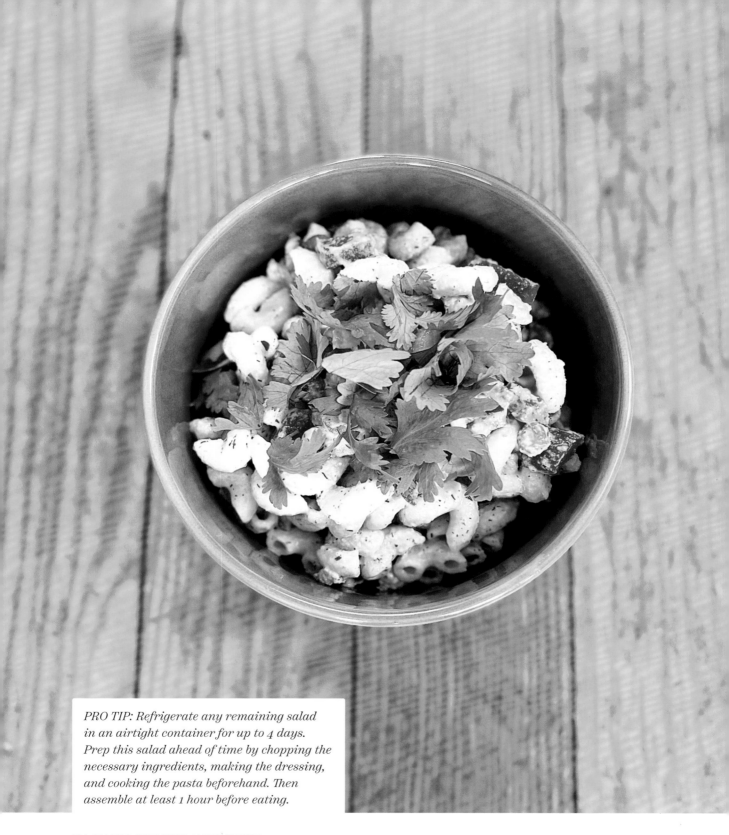

PRO TIP: Refrigerate any remaining salad in an airtight container for up to 4 days. Prep this salad ahead of time by chopping the necessary ingredients, making the dressing, and cooking the pasta beforehand. Then assemble at least 1 hour before eating.

V-MAC SALAD

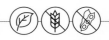

Usually I would take a hard pass on macaroni salad because many include a mayonnaise-based sauce as the primary seasoning. If, like me, you skip any dish containing mayo, take this to your next family function or work potluck—and blow people's minds that this dish is completely plant-based plus protein-dense thanks to the creamy, mayo-free dressing.

Ingredients

FOR THE DRESSING

¾ cup (75 g) raw shaved or sliced almonds

¼ cup (60 ml) water

¼ cup (60 g) Dijon mustard

3 tablespoons (45 ml) maple syrup

1 teaspoon mustard powder

FOR THE PASTA SALAD

1 box (16 ounces [454 g]) elbow macaroni or gluten-free noodles

1½ cups (255 g) frozen green peas

4 ribs celery, diced (reserve leaves for garnish)

1 large red bell pepper, diced

2 tablespoons (15 g) diced onion

2 tablespoons (8 g) dried dill

Salt, to taste

Directions

1. Start the dressing by placing the almonds and water in a saucepan and bringing to a boil. Immediately remove from the heat and let sit for 10 minutes. Drain and set aside until the pasta is done cooking.

2. Meanwhile, cook the pasta according to the package directions. Add the peas to the cooking pasta for the last few minutes of cook time.

3. Strain and rinse with cold water to ensure the pasta is completely cooled. Then drain again.

4. Transfer the pasta and peas to a large bowl. Add the celery, pepper, onion, and dill and set aside while you make the dressing.

5. Put the almonds, Dijon mustard, maple syrup, and mustard powder in a blender, pureeing until well combined.

6. Add the prepared dressing to the macaroni salad base, stirring with a large spoon until the dressing fully coats all the pasta. Add salt to taste. Eat immediately or refrigerate, covered, for 1 to 2 hours.

7. Garnish with reserved celery leaves, if desired.

YIELD 8 servings (¾ cup each)

PER SERVING 340 calories; 8 g fat; 12 g protein; 56 g carbohydrate

PREP TIME 10 mins **TOTAL TIME** 40 mins

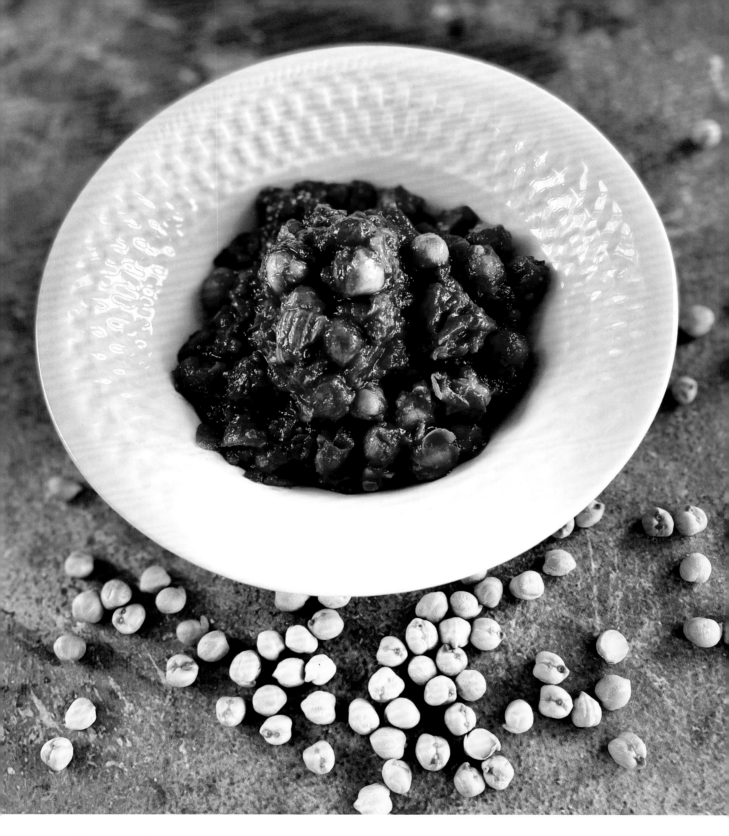

BBQ CHICKPEAS

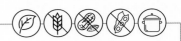

Baked beans get a remake thanks to protein-dense chickpeas in this dish. The texture may be a tad bit nuttier, but the classic BBQ flavors still make it an ideal option for picnics. These chickpeas are great served with warm bread, roasted potatoes, or Oven-Baked Apples and Kale (page 109).

Ingredients

6 cups (1.1 kg) cooked chickpeas or 3 cans (15.5 ounces [439 g]), drained and rinsed

1 can (14.5 ounces [411 g]) diced tomatoes

½ cup (120 ml) water

¼ cup (30 g) diced onion

3 tablespoons (45 ml) apple cider vinegar

2 tablespoons (30 ml) maple syrup or (43 g) honey

1 tablespoon (12 g) brown sugar

1 tablespoon (8 g) garlic powder

1 teaspoon onion powder

1 teaspoon smoked paprika

1 teaspoon salt

1 teaspoon black pepper

1 teaspoon chipotle powder

Directions

1. In a slow cooker, stir together the chickpeas, tomatoes with their juice, water, onion, vinegar, maple syrup, brown sugar, and spices.

2. Cover and cook on HIGH for 3 hours or LOW for 5 hours.

3. Add more salt, chipotle powder, or vinegar, to taste.

YIELD 6 servings (about 1 cup each)

PER SERVING 300 calories; 4 g fat; 15 g protein; 52 g carbohydrate

PREP TIME 5 mins **TOTAL TIME** 3 to 5 hours

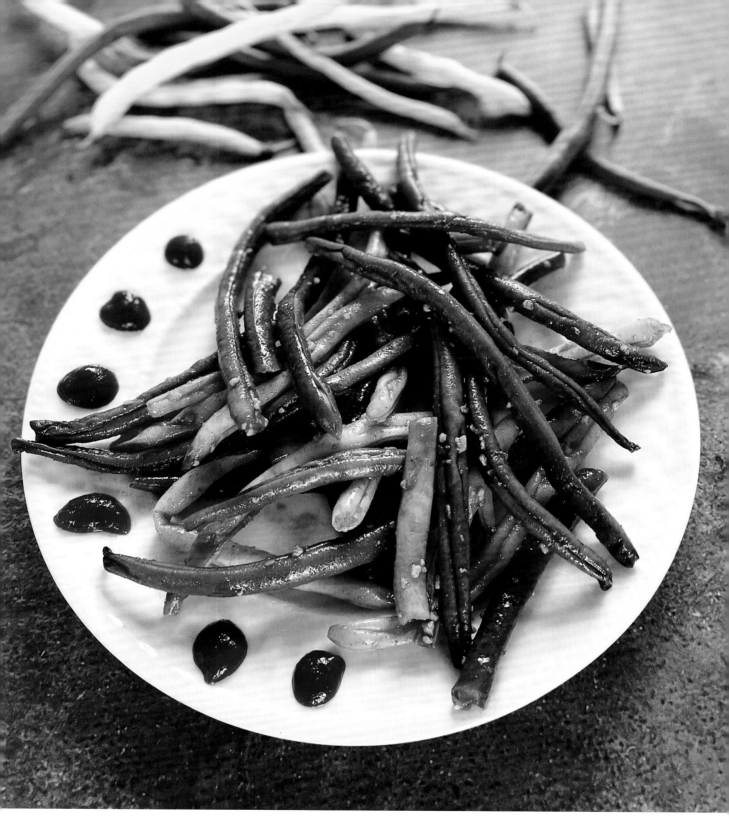

HOT GARLIC GREEN BEANS

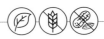

Because I adore spicy foods, this is one of those sides I could easily eat every day. It requires almost no prep work, plus it can be eaten on its own if you don't have time to make anything else. But I like to serve this with a whole grain such as brown rice or over warm udon noodles, which adds a good bump in carbs.

Ingredients

¾ lb (340 g) whole fresh green beans

½ cup (120 ml) water

2 tablespoons (30 ml) sesame oil

1 tablespoon (14 g) minced fresh ginger

2 cloves garlic, minced

2 teaspoons (5 g) ground turmeric

2 tablespoons (30 ml) rice seasoning or rice vinegar

1 tablespoon (4 g) red pepper flakes or chili garlic paste

1 tablespoon (15 ml) tamari or soy sauce

2 teaspoons (20 ml) maple syrup or agave

Directions

1. Combine the green beans and water in a large skillet over medium-high heat.

2. Cover and cook, stirring occasionally, until the beans are tender crisp, 2 to 4 minutes (you will be able to tell when their color begins to slightly change).

3. Add the sesame oil, ginger, garlic, and turmeric and cook, stirring, for 2 to 3 minutes.

4. In a small bowl, mix the rice seasoning, red pepper flakes, tamari, and maple syrup. Pour over the beans and cook for an additional 2 to 4 minutes.

> *PRO TIP Although the directions are for the stove top, you can just as easily mix all the spices and seasonings together in an oven-safe skillet or baking dish and toss in the green beans before sliding in the oven (uncovered) at 375°F (190°C, or gas mark 5) for about 15 minutes.*

YIELD 2 servings

PER SERVING 252 calories; 15 g fat; 8 g protein; 30 g carbohydrate

PREP TIME 5 mins **TOTAL TIME** 10 mins

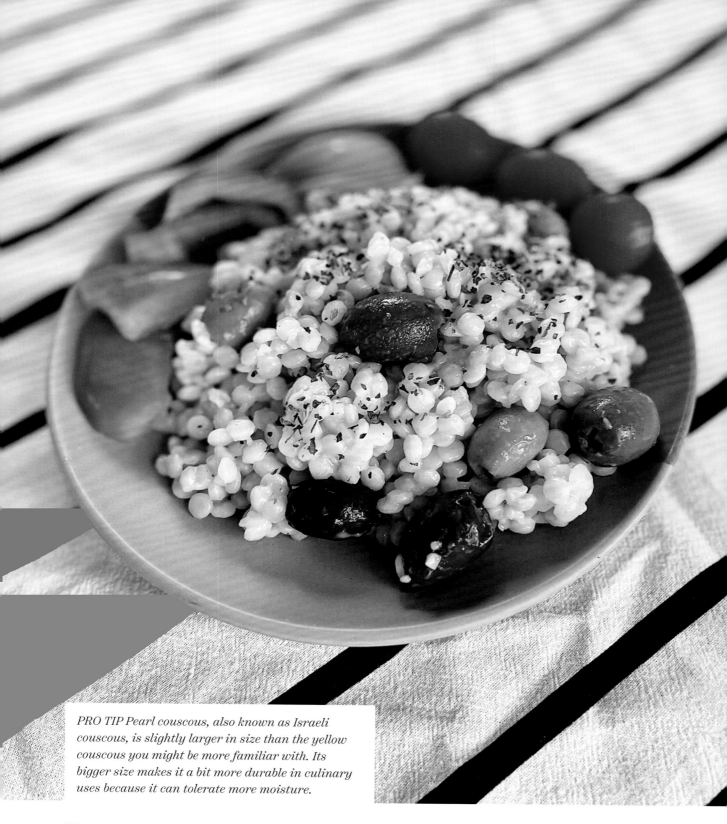

PRO TIP *Pearl couscous, also known as Israeli couscous, is slightly larger in size than the yellow couscous you might be more familiar with. Its bigger size makes it a bit more durable in culinary uses because it can tolerate more moisture.*

COCONUT LEMON COUSCOUS

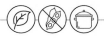

This is probably my fave dish that I experimented with during the COVID-19 pandemic while staying "safer at home." It's a cinch to make, both in terms of cost and cook time—two characteristics that guarantee a recipe gets flagged with a gold star in my recipe box.

Ingredients

2 cups (300 g) pearled couscous (see Pro Tip)

1 cup (240 ml) well-stirred coconut milk

1 teaspoon salt

1 lemon, halved

¼ cup (62 g) pitted olives (optional)

Cherry tomatoes (optional)

Strips of bell pepper (optional)

Dried oregano, for garnish

Directions

1. Prepare the couscous in a rice cooker (or on the stove top according to package directions).

2. Add the coconut milk and salt immediately after it is done cooking. Let sit for 5 minutes.

3. Lightly spritz the couscous with fresh lemon juice right before serving and add olives, tomatoes, bell pepper strips, and a shake of oregano, if desired. You can thank me later.

YIELD 4 servings (about 1 cup each)

PER SERVING 251 calories; 16 g fat; 5 g protein; 23 g carbohydrate

PREP TIME 5 mins **TOTAL TIME** 20 mins

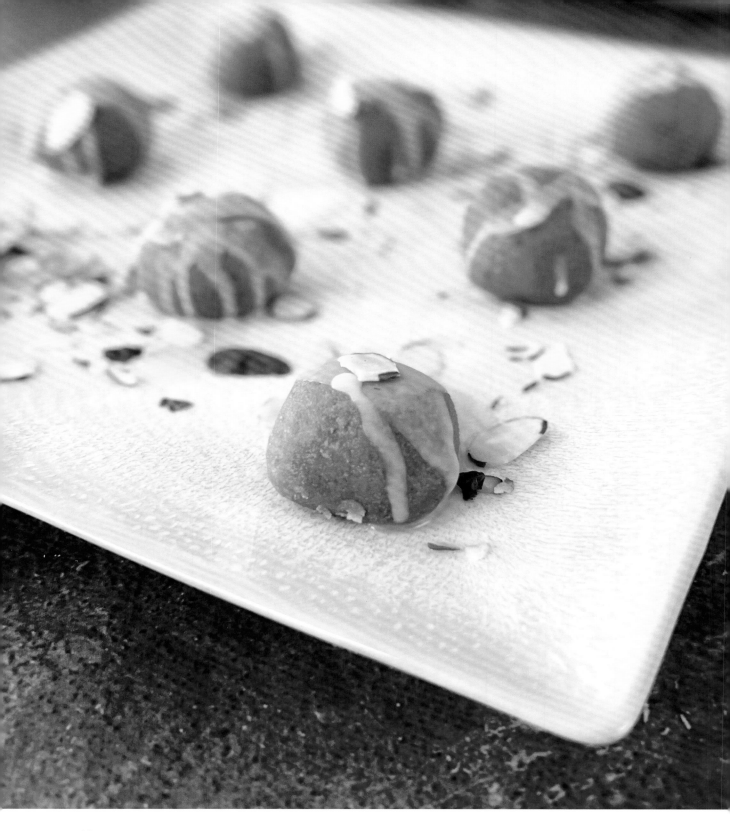

MATCHA GEMS

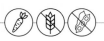

This is my rendition of Kourtney Kardashian's viral protein bites. I kick the caffeine level up in mine by adding matcha powder as a core ingredient rather than just dipping each ball into a matcha glaze, so tread lightly when tempted to pop one more gem before bedtime—but they might just be the snack you need to beat that afternoon slump, thanks to having enough protein and fat to keep you energized for longer than carb-heavy alternatives (like cookies) do.

Ingredients

1 cup (112 g) coconut flour

½ cup (128 g) nut butter

3 tablespoons (47 g) protein powder

2 tablespoons (12 g) matcha powder

2 tablespoons (30 ml) maple syrup

3 ounces (80 g) white chocolate bar (optional), coarsely chopped

2 tablespoons (16 g) shaved or sliced almonds, for garnish

Directions

1. In a bowl, stir together the coconut flour, nut butter, protein and matcha powders, and maple syrup until smooth.

2. Roll out small spoonfuls of the dough into 10 small balls ("gems") and set them on a parchment- or waxed paper–lined plate or baking dish.

3. Freeze the balls for at least 30 minutes.

4. When the balls are frozen, put the chocolate in a microwave-safe bowl and heat on high 45 seconds to 1 minute, stirring half-way through. (Stop when most of the chocolate is melted, then stir until completely melted.) Immediately drizzle the melted chocolate over the gems.

5. Put the gems back in the freezer for 5 to 10 minutes so the chocolate can set.

6. Sprinkle with the shaved almonds, if desired, before eating.

> *PRO TIP Remember to carefully scan the ingredient label of protein powders if it's essential the kind you use be free of dairy, soy, or nuts.*

YIELD 10 servings (1 gem each)

PER SERVING 173 calories; 12 g fat; 4 g protein; 18 g carbohydrate

PREP TIME 20 mins **TOTAL TIME** 1 hour

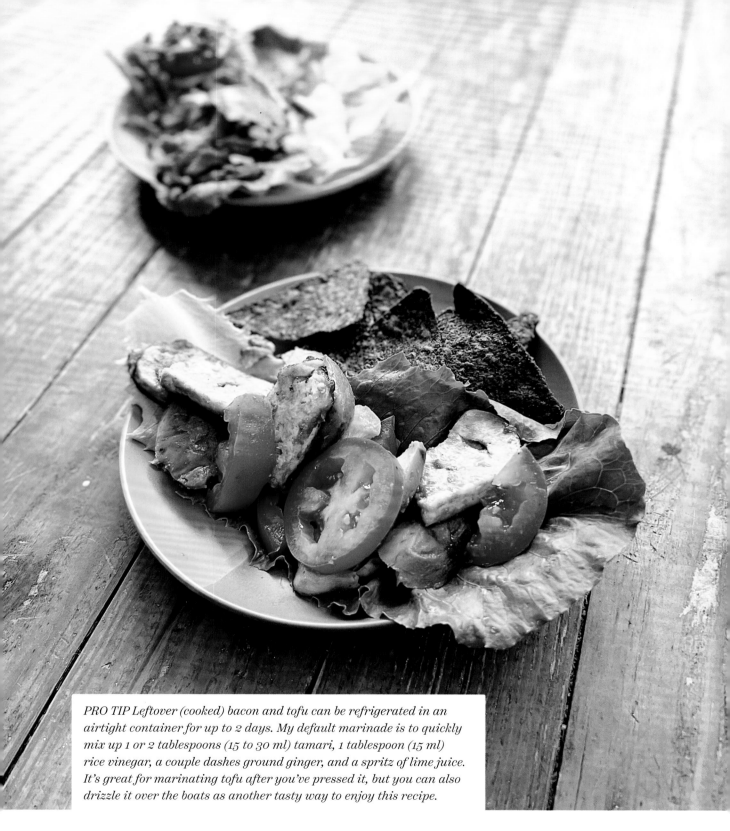

PRO TIP Leftover (cooked) bacon and tofu can be refrigerated in an airtight container for up to 2 days. My default marinade is to quickly mix up 1 or 2 tablespoons (15 to 30 ml) tamari, 1 tablespoon (15 ml) rice vinegar, a couple dashes ground ginger, and a spritz of lime juice. It's great for marinating tofu after you've pressed it, but you can also drizzle it over the boats as another tasty way to enjoy this recipe.

BLT (& TLT) BOATS

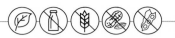

Turns out bacon, lettuce, and tomato is quite a tasty combo even without the bread. And if you're vegan and/or kosher, *tofu*, lettuce, and tomato is an equally yummy alternative. You'll enjoy eating either of these protein-based snacks much more than a chalky power bar. Plus, they're easy to pack-up as a "grab and go" for longer days at the office or on road trips. (Wait to assemble each boat until ready to eat.)

Ingredients

Nonstick cooking spray or olive oil

1 package (14 ounces [396 g]) firm tofu, drained (see Pro Tip)

6 slices bacon

8 romaine lettuce leaves

2 or 3 plum tomatoes, sliced

1 large avocado, diced or sliced

¼ cup (60 ml) fresh lime juice

1 teaspoon freshly ground black pepper

Salt, to taste

Directions

1. Preheat the oven to 400°F (200°C, or gas mark 6). Spray a baking sheet with nonstick cooking spray (or lightly coat with olive oil).

2. If making the TLT version, press the tofu for at least 10 minutes before slicing, crosswise, into 10 to 12 slabs. (If you don't have a tofu press, refer to the Pro Tip in Faux Fried Tofu on page 69.)

3. Lay the sliced tofu or bacon (if making the BLT version) on the baking sheet in a single layer. (Be sure to use separate trays if preparing this meal for meat eaters and vegetarians.) Flip everything over once before putting in the oven.

4. Bake until the tofu is golden brown and/or the bacon is deep golden brown and crispy, 10 to 20 minutes. Check every couple of minutes, to avoid overcooking either the bacon or tofu.

5. Remove from the oven and let cool before chopping or crumbling the bacon.

6. Fill each lettuce leaf with bacon or slices of tofu, tomatoes, and avocado. Drizzle with lime juice, and sprinkle with pepper and salt.

YIELD 4 servings

PER SERVING (tofu) 237 calories; 17 g fat; 13 g protein; 14 g carbohydrate

PER SERVING (bacon) 215 calories; 13 g fat; 15 g protein; 14 g carbohydrate

PREP TIME 10 mins **TOTAL TIME** 30 mins

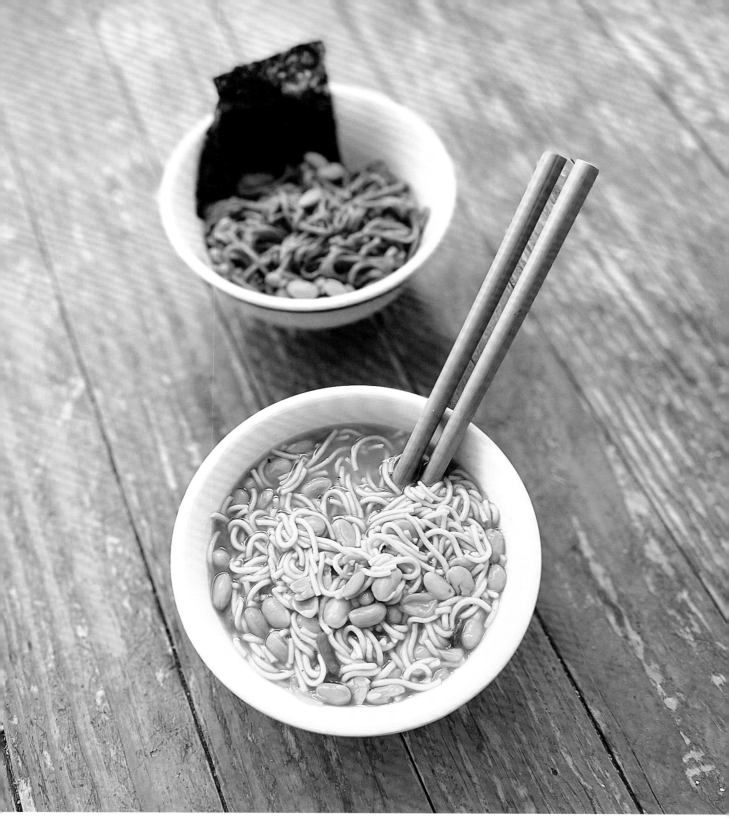

BOUGIE RAMEN

For many of us, instant ramen was in steady rotation during our adolescent or college years. So much so that it's one of the foods I most often hear people reference having a sudden craving for—including colleagues in the fitness industry who are known to almost never take nutritional shortcuts. However, it's hard to let go of cheap food we enjoy that takes very little time to prepare. And thanks to this DIY version that's much lower in sodium—*and* actually includes more than one food group—now you don't have to.

Ingredients

1 bundle soba noodles or udon noodles (⅓ package) or 1 packet instant ramen noodles (discard spice packet)

¼ cup (28 g) shelled edamame (fresh or thawed from frozen)

1 tablespoon (15 ml) tamari or soy sauce

2 teaspoons (5 g) ground ginger

1 to 2 cups (235 to 470 ml) vegetable broth, warmed (optional)

1 tablespoon (15 ml) fresh lime juice

Directions

1. Cook the noodles according to the package directions.

2. Meanwhile, stir-fry the edamame in a small skillet sprayed with a nonstick oil spray.

3. Drain and rinse the noodles when done, then add to the edamame.

4. Stir in the tamari and ginger.

5. If you want to savor the ramen as a soup, slowly add the veggie broth until you reach your desired amount of soup base. Or simply savor it as a noodle dish!

6. Stir in the lime juice then carefully transfer to a soup bowl before digging in.

YIELD 1 serving

PER SERVING 373 calories; 3 g fat; 19 g protein; 75 g carbohydrate

PREP TIME 5 mins **TOTAL TIME** 15 mins

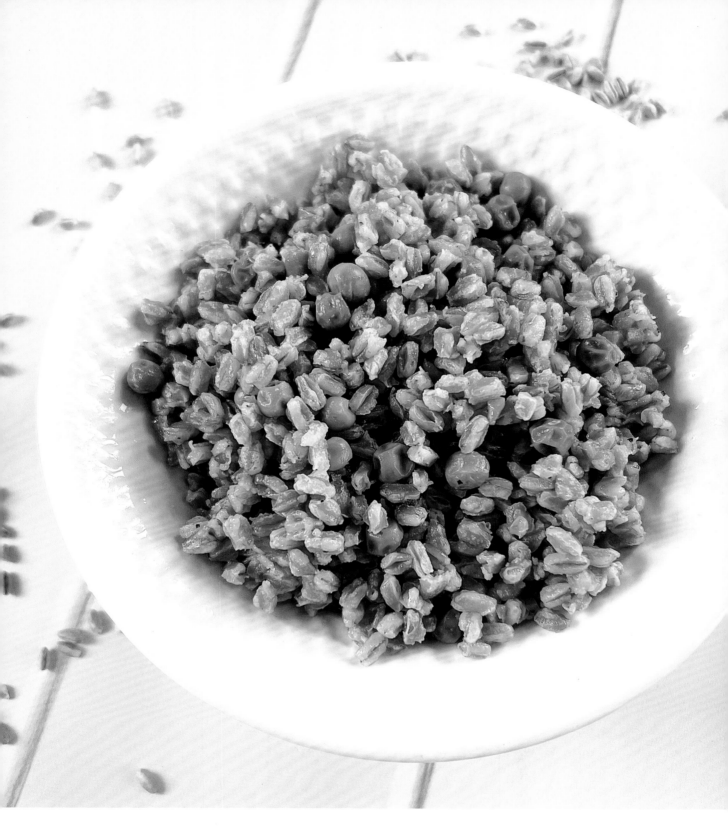

SESAME FARRO

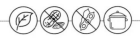

I'll admit this recipe is *very* simple, but food doesn't need to be complex or time-consuming to be good. This is the snack to make when you want a savory nosh *now*. It also makes a yummy side to a precooked protein source if you've got 15 minutes or less to get dinner on the table. Lastly, omit the peas or sub in frozen kale and pair this dish with eggs for a quick breakfast bowl option.

Ingredients

2 cups (360 g) farro

¾ cup (128 g) frozen peas

2 tablespoons (30 ml) toasted sesame oil

1 tablespoon (15 ml) fresh lemon juice

2 teaspoons (9 g) minced garlic

Directions

1. Cook the farro according to the package directions in a rice cooker or on the stove top.

2. Add in the peas in the last 10 minutes of cooking.

3. Once the farro is cooked, drain any excess water.

4. Mix in the sesame oil, lemon juice, and garlic. Enjoy warm or cold.

PRO TIP Sesame Farro can be refrigerated in an airtight container for up to 3 days.

YIELD 4 servings

PER SERVING 361 calories; 7 g fat; 13 g protein; 64 g carbohydrate

PREP TIME 5 mins **TOTAL TIME** 15 mins

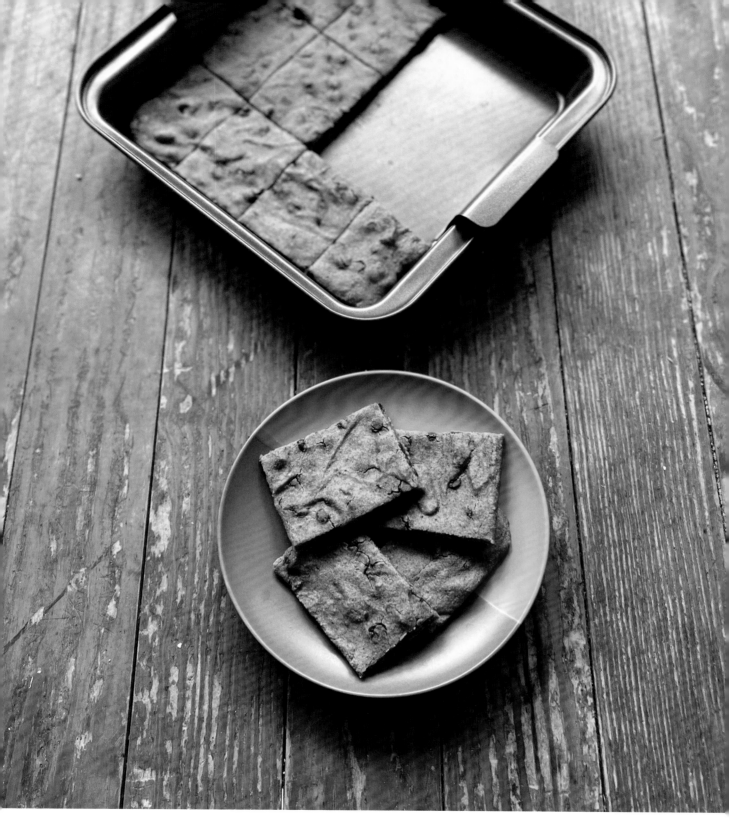

PUMPKIN OAT BARS

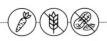

I feel like pumpkin-flavored beverages and food have been trending for about a decade now. And their popularity doesn't seem to be waning anytime soon. So if you adore the lattes, here's my version of a pumpkin spice bar that'll keep you going longer than that PSL.

Ingredients

Nonstick cooking spray

1 cup (244 g) pumpkin puree

½ cup (120 ml) maple syrup

½ cup (128 g) natural creamy nut butter

2 large eggs (or equivalent egg substitute)

2 teaspoons (10 ml) vanilla extract

½ cup (62 g) oat flour

¼ cup (28 g) coconut flour

2 teaspoons (5 g) ground cinnamon

2 teaspoons (5 g) ground allspice

¼ teaspoon baking powder

¼ teaspoon salt (if using unsalted nut butter, increase to ½ teaspoon salt)

½ cup (125 g) mini chocolate chips (or caramel or butterscotch)

Directions

1. Preheat the oven to 350°F (180°C, or gas mark 4). Lightly grease an 8-inch (20-cm) square baking pan with nonstick cooking spray.

2. In a medium bowl, combine the pumpkin, maple syrup, nut butter, eggs, and vanilla. Whisk until smooth.

3. In a separate bowl, stir together the flours, cinnamon, allspice, baking powder, and salt. Pour the wet ingredients into the bowl with the dry ingredients and mix until well combined.

4. Fold in the chocolate chips using a spatula, and then evenly spread the mixture into the prepared baking dish.

5. Bake until a toothpick inserted into the center comes out mostly clean, 25 to 30 minutes.

6. Let cool in the pan before cutting into 12 squares.

PRO TIP Store leftovers in the fridge for up to 3 days. Warm for 15 seconds in the microwave before eating. Can also be kept frozen for up to 2 months. And if you or anyone in your household has a nut allergy, simply use sunflower butter in place of the nut butter, plus omit the coconut flour by using more oat flour instead.

YIELD 12 servings

PER SERVING 166 calories; 10 g fat; 4 g protein; 17 g carbohydrate

PREP TIME 10 mins **TOTAL TIME** 45 mins·

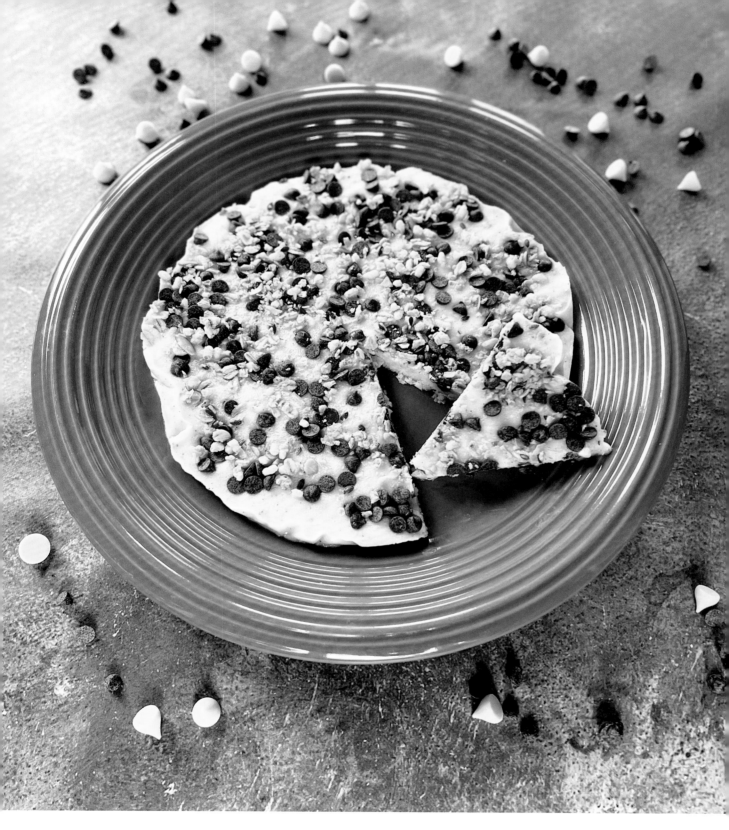

DARK CHOCOLATE YOGURT BARK

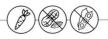

People went bananas when yogurt bark started popping up on Instagram and TikTok. And I get why. It's hard not to fall hard for a "sweet treat" that's super easy to make, is packed with protein, and is low cal.

Ingredients

3 cups (680 g) plain full-fat Greek yogurt or nondairy yogurt

⅓ cup (113 g) agave or honey

1 teaspoon vanilla extract

¾ cup (105 g) granola

¼ cup (62 g) dark chocolate chips

Directions

1. Line an 8-inch (20-cm) round cake pan (or square baking dish) with parchment paper or aluminum foil.

2. In a medium bowl, stir together the yogurt, agave, and vanilla.

3. Pour into the dish and spread in an even layer.

4. Top with the granola and dark chocolate chips, plus other toppings of your choice (see Pro Tip).

5. Freeze for at least 2 hours. To serve, lift out the bark and cut into 8 pieces.

> *PRO TIP Other topping ideas include strawberries, peanut butter, crushed almonds, or pistachios. Bark can be kept frozen in a sealed container for up to 2 weeks.*

YIELD 8 servings

PER SERVING 171 calories; 5 g fat; 9 g protein; 22 g carbohydrate

PREP TIME 10 mins **TOTAL TIME** 2.25 hours

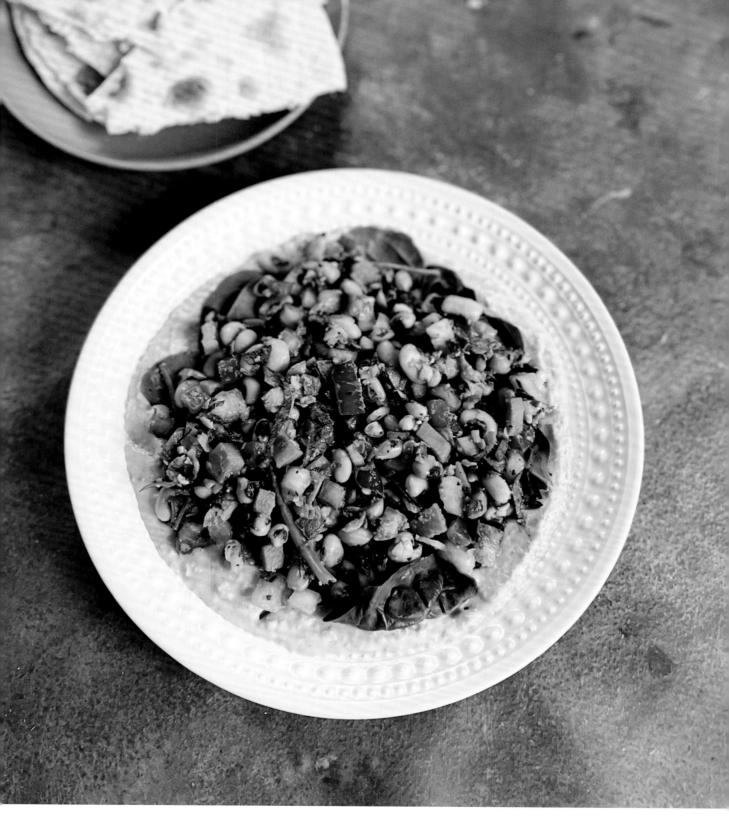

SOUTHERN HUMMUS PLATE

Southern food frequently gets a bad rap for being unhealthy, despite homegrown foods being an attribute to this type of cuisine. If you're a hobby farmer or the type of green thumb that has a makeshift balcony garden in the city, here's a new idea on what to do with those veggies you're growing by using them in an energizing snack.

Ingredients

1 cup (260 g) cooked or canned, drained, and rinsed black-eyed peas

¼ cup (30 g) diced red onion

1 small red bell pepper, diced

1 small carrot, diced

1 rib celery, diced

2 tablespoons (30 ml) balsamic vinegar

1 tablespoon (15 ml) olive oil

2 teaspoons (8 g) dried dill

1 teaspoon kosher salt

1 teaspoon black pepper

1 cup (224 g) prepared hummus

1 cup (28 g) fresh spinach

Warm pita bread wedges or tortilla chips, for serving

Directions

1. In a medium bowl, stir together the black-eyed peas, onion, bell pepper, carrot, celery, vinegar, oil, dill, salt, and black pepper. Chill for at least 10 minutes.

2. Use a spatula or the back of spoon to spread the hummus onto a large plate.

3. Layer the spinach on the hummus.

4. Top with the black-eyed-pea salad, making sure to evenly cover the hummus and spinach base.

5. Enjoy with warm pita or tortilla chips.

YIELD 4 servings

PER SERVING 212 calories; 9 g fat; 7 g protein; 26 g carbohydrate

PREP TIME 20 mins **TOTAL TIME** 30 mins

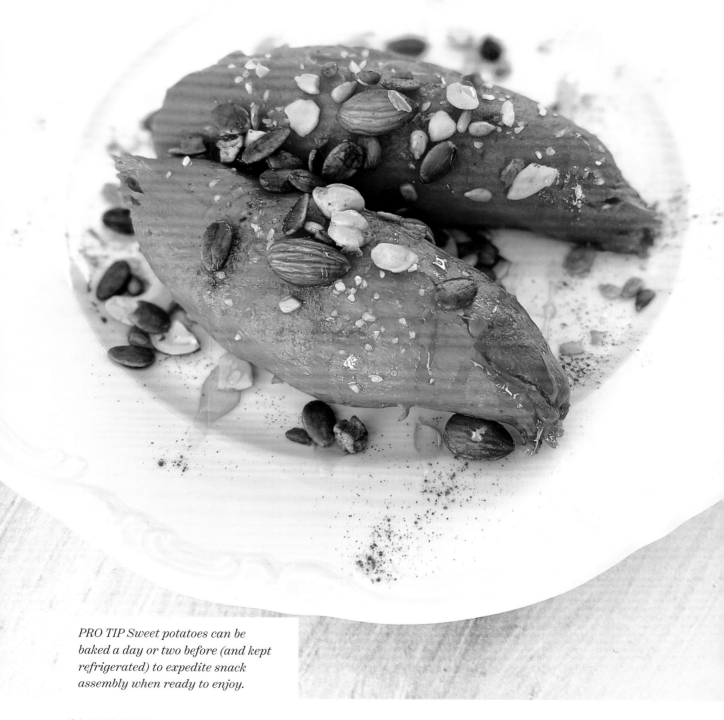

PRO TIP Sweet potatoes can be baked a day or two before (and kept refrigerated) to expedite snack assembly when ready to enjoy.

CINNAMON BATATAS

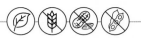

I rarely skip breakfast. But on those occasions when I do, I usually need a heartier nosh in the late afternoon. Especially if I know dinner won't be ready until an hour (or two) post sunset. Thus, these batatas (Spanish for "sweet potato") quench hunger well enough to help me stay focused mentally, plus squeeze in an early evening run, on days when my food intake start off rocky.

Ingredients

Two sweet potatoes (about 8 ounces [227 g] each), washed and patted dry

¼ cup (62 g) chopped nuts or seeds

2 tablespoons (43 g) agave or honey

1 tablespoon (8 g) ground cinnamon

1 teaspoon kosher salt

Directions

1. Preheat the oven to 400°F (200°C, or gas mark 6).

2. Poke holes into each potato with a fork.

3. Place the potatoes on a baking sheet and roast until tender, about 40 minutes.

4. Remove from the oven and cool for 3 to 5 minutes before carefully removing the outer peel.

5. To serve, put each potato on a plate and top with the nuts, agave, cinnamon, and salt.

YIELD 2 servings

PER SERVING 295 calories; 9 g fat; 6 g protein; 52 g carbohydrate

PREP TIME 5 mins **TOTAL TIME** 50 mins

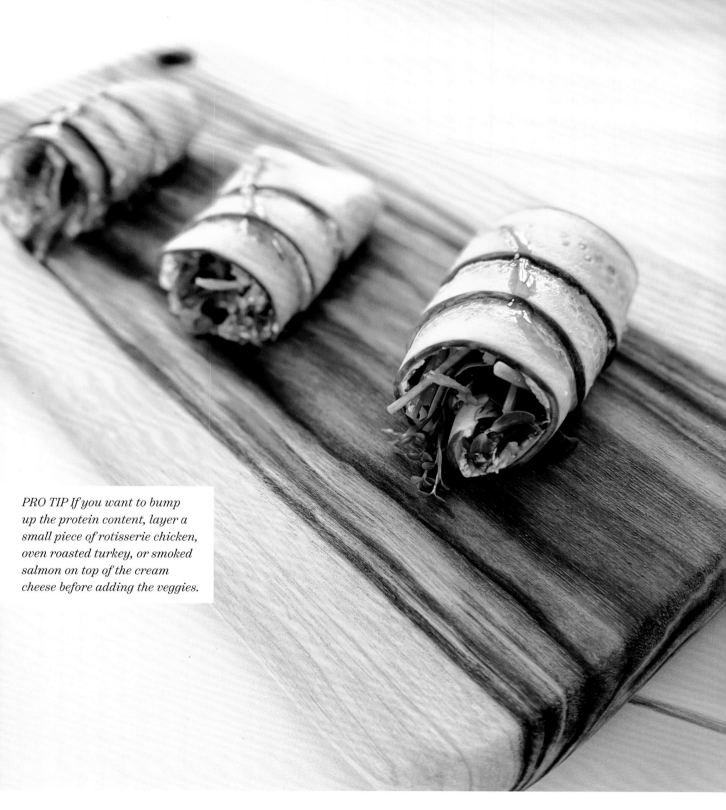

PRO TIP If you want to bump up the protein content, layer a small piece of rotisserie chicken, oven roasted turkey, or smoked salmon on top of the cream cheese before adding the veggies.

CUCUMBER ROLLS

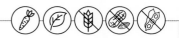

The only reason I don't eat these rolls every day is that I don't always have all the fresh ingredients on hand. The plating. The texture. The light drizzle of Thai Sweet Chili Sauce. The combination earns the descriptor of "crave-worthy" on every level. Start stocking up on cucumbers because you're about to fall in love.

Ingredients

2 large seedless cucumbers, cut in half lengthwise

6 tablespoons (90 g) cream cheese or vegan cream cheese, preferably herb-flavored (or add your own)

1 cup (35 g) alfalfa sprouts

½ cup (57 g) shredded carrots

½ cup (14 g) fresh spinach

Thai chili sauce or sweet and sour sauce, for serving

Directions

1. Starting on the cut side of each cucumber half, use a mandolin to thinly slice the cucumbers lengthwise.

2. Put 1 cucumber slice on a cutting board or plate, then spread a thin layer of cream cheese on it. Layer a another (slightly shorter) piece on top of it before also putting cream cheese on the second strip. Add a third (slightly shorter strip) on top of that one when done.

3. Divide the sprouts, carrots, and spinach into 6 equal portions. Place a portion of each veggie on top of the layered cucumber slices, crosswise, then gently roll together. Set on a cutting board or serving plate, seam-side down.

4. Repeat using the remaining ingredients.

5. Serve with one or both sauces, as desired.

YIELD 2 servings (3 rolls each)

PER SERVING 172 calories; 11 g fat; 6 g protein; 13 g carbohydrate

PREP TIME 25 mins **TOTAL TIME** 25 mins

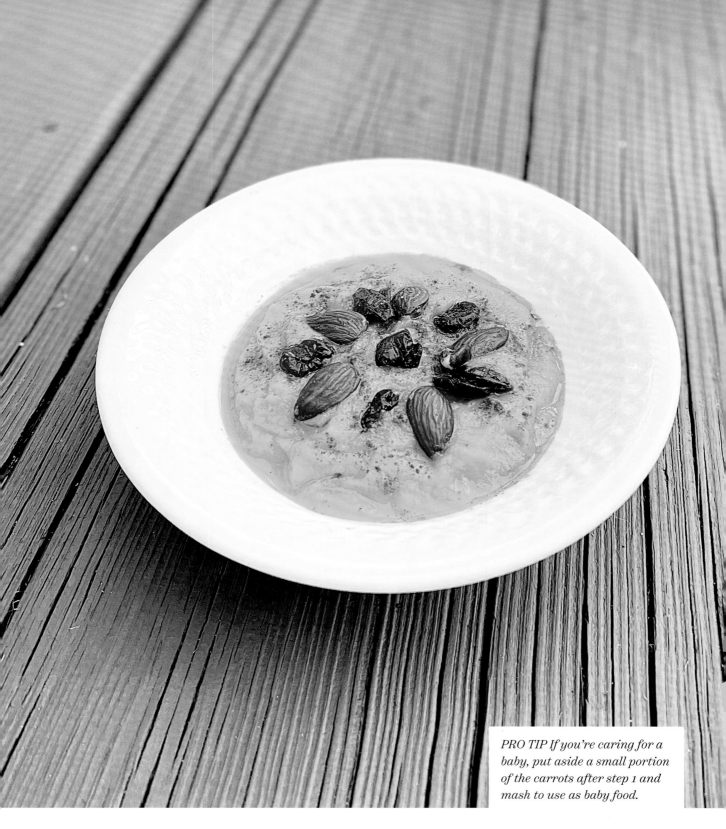

GAJAR HALWA

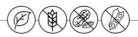

This dish is a rare sweet treat that's allowed during certain seasons for those doing a detox-focused meal plan centered in ayurvedic philosophy, which is how I first came to try it. Gajar Halwa is a dish that originates from Arabic and Indian cultures. It is made primarily of carrots and gets an extra boost of sweetness thanks to the dried fruit, although the density of the final product is attributable to the thickening and creaminess of the milk.

Ingredients

10 to 12 medium carrots, grated

1 cup (235 ml) vegetable broth

½ cup (120 ml) maple syrup

3 tablespoons (24 g) ground cinnamon

1 tablespoon (8 g) ground cumin

1 cup (240 ml) well-stirred coconut milk or whole milk

4 teaspoons (16 g) dried cranberries or raisins

2 tablespoons (16 g) whole or shaved almonds (optional)

Directions

1. In a large saucepan over low heat, combine the carrots and broth. Keep over low until the carrots are cooked, 15 to 20 minutes.

2. Add the maple syrup, cinnamon, and cumin. Gradually increase the heat to medium, stirring frequently to keep the carrots from sticking to the pan.

3. Once the carrots are completely tender, remove from the heat and cool for 8 to 10 minutes.

4. Transfer to a mixing bowl, then add the coconut milk. Use a fork or the back of a large spoon to mash, then mix, the milk into the carrots.

5. Garnish each serving with 1 teaspoon cranberries, ½ tablespoon almonds (if using), and an extra dash of cinnamon, if desired. Enjoy while still warm.

YIELD 4 servings (about 1 cup each)

PER SERVING 269 calories; 16 g fat; 3 g protein; 33 g carbohydrate

PREP TIME 15 mins **TOTAL TIME** 45 mins

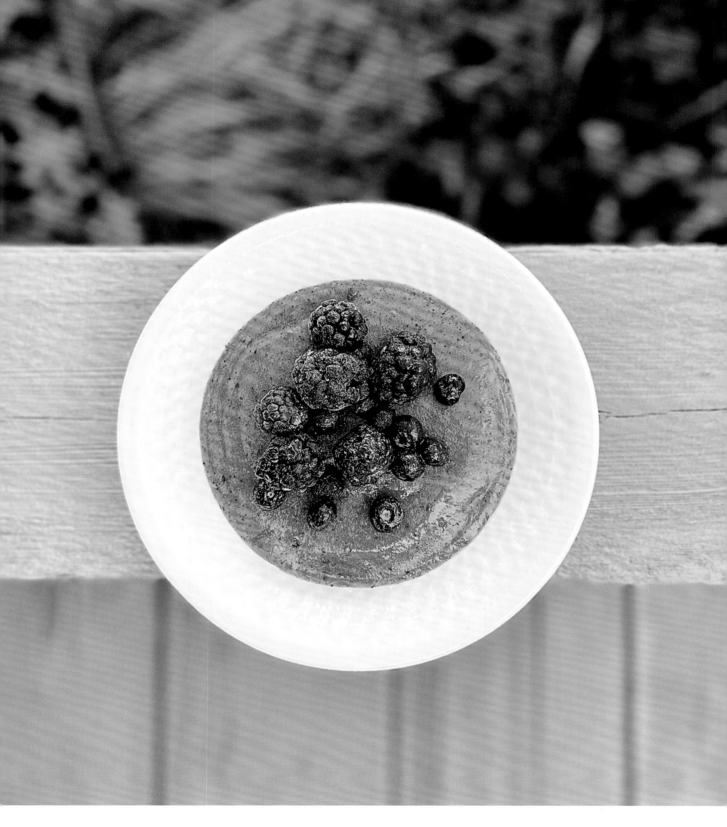

WILD BERRY FRO-YO

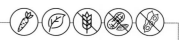

One of my biggest "pleasure foods" is probably frozen desserts. *Cold* and *sweet* are quite a seductive pair. It's also why my general rule of thumb is not to keep too many goodies tucked away in the freezer. That way, if I really want an edible treat, I have to make it. Hope you end up adoring this immediate craving cure as much as I do.

Ingredients

2 cups (454 g) vanilla Greek yogurt or nondairy yogurt

1½ cups (222 g) frozen mixed berries + additional, for garnish

1 tablespoon (21 g) agave or honey

¼ cup (54 g) ice (optional)

2 tablespoons (31 g) protein powder (optional)

2 teaspoons (5 g) cane sugar, for garnish

Directions

1. Combine the yogurt, berries, and agave in a blender or food processor and blend until it comes together in a smooth ice cream–like texture, about 25 seconds.

2. If adding ice and/or protein powder, blend for another 15 seconds. Either way, be sure all the berries have been fully blended. Restart for an additional 10 seconds if not.

3. Divide this berry yogurt "base" between 2 bowls and place in the freezer for at least 25 minutes so it can harden. Take the bowls out when ready to eat.

4. Serve, if desired, with additional frozen berries and a sprinkle of cane sugar on top.

YIELD 2 servings

PER SERVING 334 calories; 7 g fat; 20 g protein; 53 g carbohydrate

PREP TIME 5 mins **TOTAL TIME** 30 mins

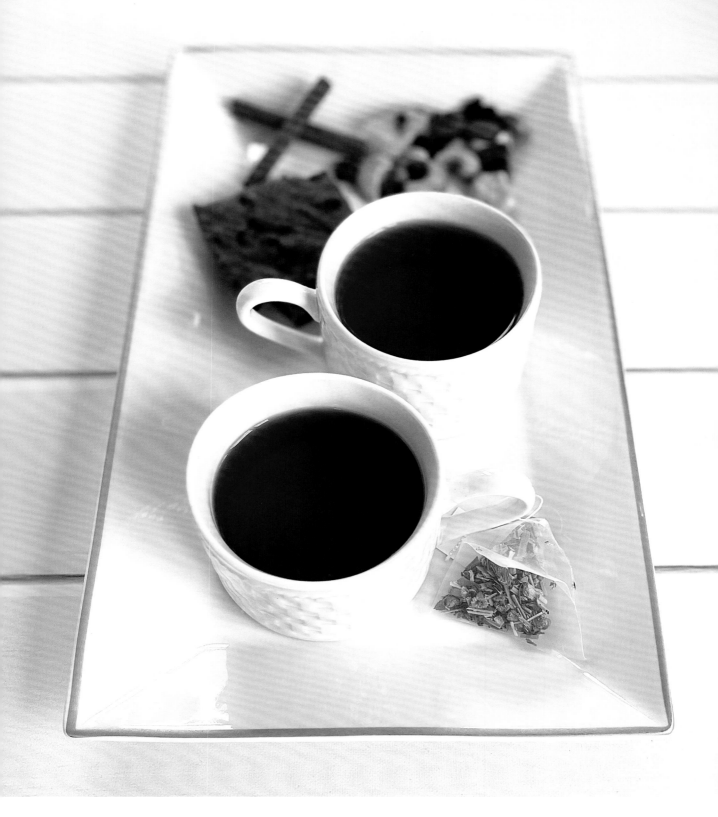

S-N-S TODDY

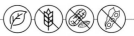

The "S-n-S" stands for sugar and spice—a contemporary moniker I'm bestowing on a classic sip. This drink is a stellar choice on evenings when you're craving an alcohol-free nightcap. And because it is boozeless, there's really no good reason not to have a second round.

Ingredients

3 cups (700 ml) water

2 Sweet and Spicy or orange spice tea bags

2 teaspoons (20 ml) maple syrup or (14 g) honey

2 teaspoons (10 ml) fresh lemon juice (or to taste)

1 to 1½ teaspoons (4 g) ground cloves

2 or 3 cinnamon sticks

2 or 3 lemon slices (optional)

Directions

1. Bring the water to a high simmer in an electric kettle or teapot on the stove top. Remove from the heat source, add the teabags, and steep for 3 to 4 minutes.

2. Equally divide the maple syrup, lemon juice, cloves, and cinnamon sticks between 2 or 3 mugs.

3. Pour the tea into the mugs, stirring each until the maple syrup is blended. Use the lemon slices for an extra burst of citrus, or as an edible adornment, if desired.

YIELD 2 or 3 servings

PER SERVING 17 calories; 0 g fat; 0 g protein; 5 g carbohydrate

PREP TIME 5 mins **TOTAL TIME** 10 mins

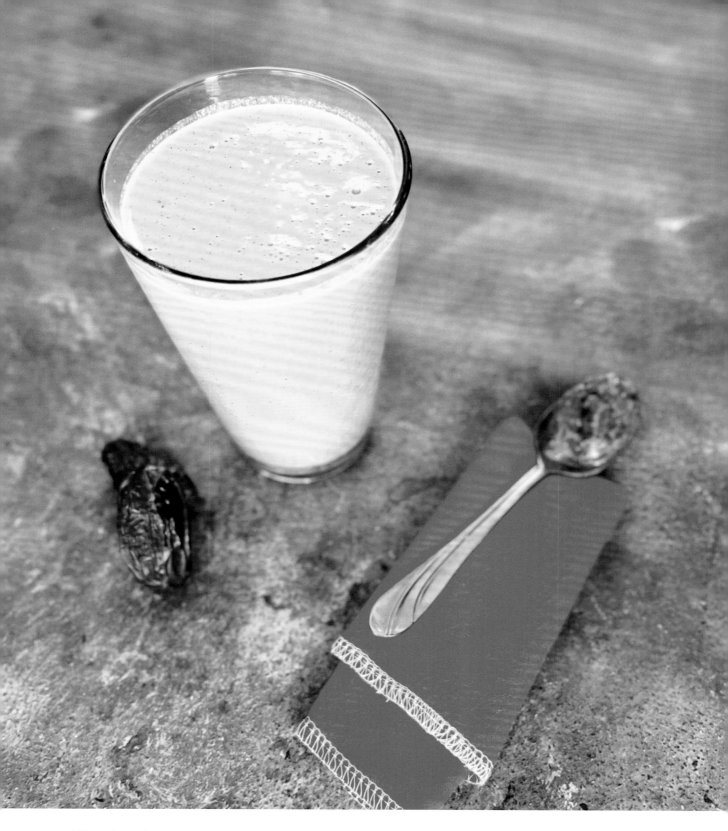

PB BOOST

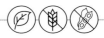

A protein smoothie is one of the quickest and most low-maintenance nosh options to hit your daily target for protein. On average, I have at least three of these a week because they're so tasty and keep me on track ratio-wise for the week.

Ingredients

1 cup (235 ml) whole or oat milk

½ cup (74 g) frozen banana pieces

¼ cup (64 g) peanut butter

2 pitted dates

2 tablespoons (31 g) protein powder

1 tablespoon (21 g) agave or honey

½ teaspoon ground cinnamon

Directions

To a blender, add the milk, bananas, peanut butter, dates, protein powder, agave, and cinnamon. Blend on high speed until smooth consistency. (If the shake is too thick, add a little more milk or ice cubes. Blend again until everything is well combined.) Pour the shake into a glass—and sip slowly.

YIELD 1 serving

PER SERVING 781 calories; 37 g fat; 25 g protein; 108 g carbohydrate

PREP TIME 5 mins **TOTAL TIME** 5 mins

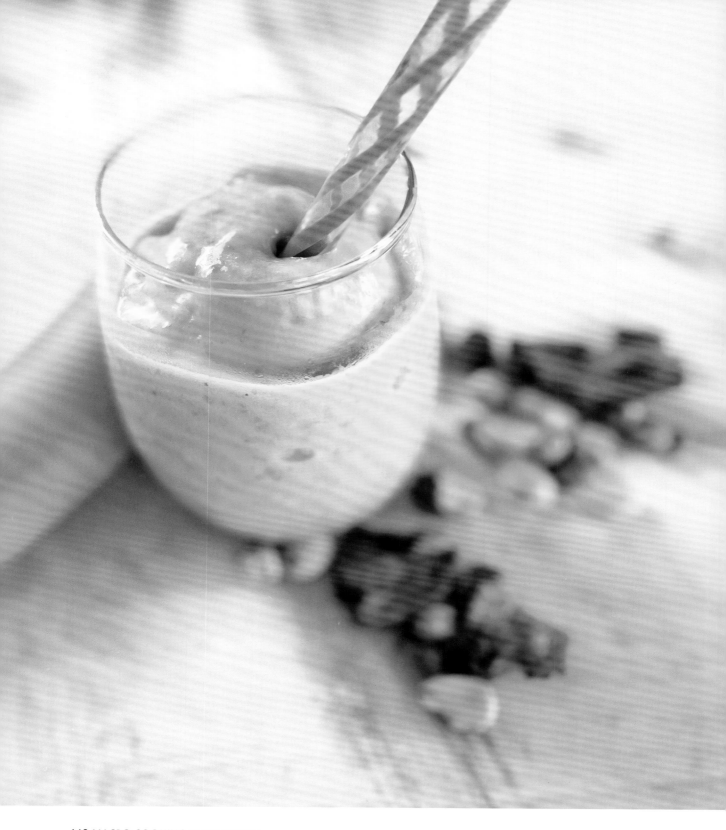

LOW-CAL LASSI

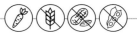

When I'm hanging lakeside or hosting a summer soirée, my preference is to drink *mindfully* by mixing up an inventive adult beverage sans alcohol, like this one that is just as delectable as a piña colada or other frozen cocktail that's loaded with calories—yet much less nutritious.

Ingredients

2 cups (510 g) plain nonfat yogurt

1½ cups (222 g) frozen mango chunks

½ cup (120 ml) almond milk or milk of choice

2 tablespoons (43 g) honey or agave

1 tablespoon (8 g) ground cinnamon

2 tablespoons (28 g) ground flaxseed (optional)

Directions

Using a blender or food processer, puree the yogurt, mango, almond milk, honey, cinnamon, and flax, if using. Divide between 2 glasses and promptly enjoy or refrigerate for up to 1 hour before serving.

YIELD 2 servings

PER SERVING 323 calories; 2 g fat; 22 g protein; 59 g carbohydrate

PREP TIME 5 mins **TOTAL TIME** 10 mins

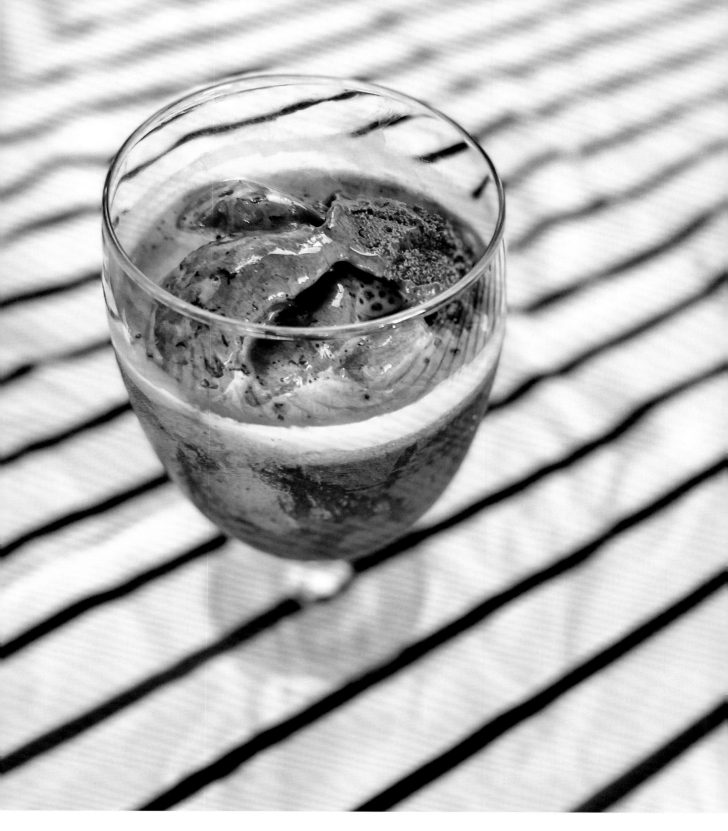

MOCHA AFFOGATO

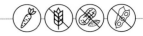

Translated into English from Italian, the word *affogato* means "drowned," which I choose to interpret as explicit permission to do a heavy pour of espresso. Even if you decide to stick to one shot, you'll still detect notes of *bitter* and *sweet* in each bite. This is a decadent treat meant to be enjoyed day or night.

Ingredients

1 shot espresso or ½ cup (120 ml) freshly brewed strong coffee

½ cup (75 g) dark chocolate ice cream or gelato

1 teaspoon cacao nibs, for garnish

Directions

1. Using your desired brewing method, brew 1 shot espresso (or coffee).

2. While the coffee brews, put the ice cream into a drinking glass or large coffee mug.

3. Pour the hot espresso (or coffee) over the ice cream.

4. Top with cacao nibs, if using, and enjoy immediately.

YIELD 1 serving

PER SERVING 220 calories; 15 g fat; 4 g protein; 22 g carbohydrate

PREP TIME 5 mins **TOTAL TIME** 10 mins

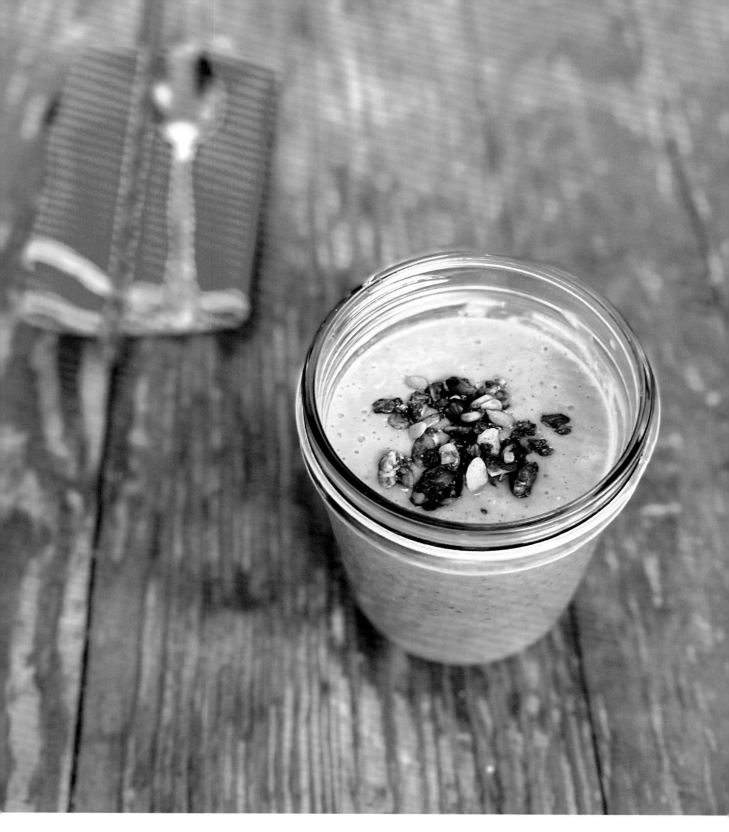

GREEN TEA SMOOTHIE

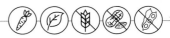

Full confession: I am not a *green* smoothie girl. A year ago, the typical smoothie I made consisted of bananas, almond milk, and maybe, a few dashes of cinnamon. But figuring out how to infuse a natural caffeine boost—while also significantly elevating the nutrient content of a single serving—finally awakened me to the many benefits of pairing leafy greens with their fruity cousins in a single glass.

Ingredients

1 frozen banana (or ¼ cup [40 g] frozen pineapple)

½ cup (120 ml) brewed green tea, cooled

½ cup (120 ml) low-fat milk, cashew milk, or coconut milk creamer

3 small slices avocado

3 or 4 small kale leaves

1 to 2 teaspoons honey or agave syrup

1 to 2 teaspoons granola, for garnish

Directions

In a blender, combine the banana, tea, milk, avocado, kale, and honey. Blend until the desired consistency is reached. Pour into a chilled glass, garnish with granola (if desired), and raise the glass in "cheers" to the day ahead!

YIELD 1 serving

PER SERVING 213 calories; 9 g fat; 4 g protein; 32 g carbohydrate

PREP TIME 10 mins **TOTAL TIME** 15 mins

BIBLIOGRAPHY

American College of Sports Medicine. "Protein Intake for Optimal Muscle Maintenance" (2015).

American Heart Association. "Protein and Heart Health" (March 26, 2017).

American Heart Association. "Trans Fats" (March 23, 2017).

Dunford, Marie and J. Andrew Doyle. *Nutrition for Sport and Exercise*, 4th ed. Boston, MA: Cengage, 2019

GBD 2017 Diet Collaborators. "Health effects of dietary risks in 195 countries, 1990–2017: A systematic analysis for the Global Burden of Disease Study 2017." *The Lancet* (April 3, 2019).

Hass, Elson M. and Buck Levin. *Staying Healthy with Nutrition: The Complete Guide to Diet and Nutritional Medicine*. Berkeley, CA: Celestial Arts, 2006.

Mangels, Reed, Virginia Messina, and Mark Messina. *The Dietitian's Guide to Vegetarian Diets: Issues and Applications*, 3rd ed. Burlington, MA: Jones & Bartlett Learning, 2010.

Research and Markets. "Global Weight Loss Products and Services Market Report 2021: The Business of Weight Loss in the 20th and 21st Centuries" (July 2021).

INDEX

ABOUT THE AUTHOR

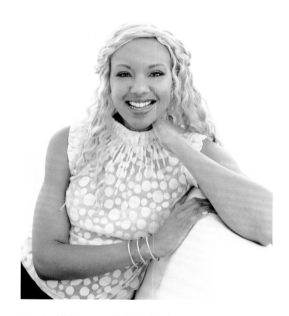

Rachel Werner, C.H.N. is the Nutrition and Fitness editor for TOPS (Take off Pounds Sensibly) and has contributed print and photography content to TheKitchn, The Spruce Eats, The Gourmet Insider, Fabulous Wisconsin, Entrepreneurial Chef, and *Hobby Farms* magazine. A selection of Rachel's recipes are also included in the book *Wisconsin Cocktails*. She is a Certified Holistic Nutritionist as well as a certified yoga instructor and mindfulness practitioner. She resides in Madison, WI.
Follow her on Instagram @therealscript and @trulyplanted or Twitter @therealscripts.